DATE DUE

FEB 2 1 1995		
MAY 2 0 1996		
MAY 1 5		
OCT 3 0 2000		
NOV 2 0 2000		
MAR 2 5 2002		

DEMCO 38-297

YOUR
SKIN
From Acne to Zits

JEROME Z. LITT, M.D.

DEMBNER BOOKS • New York

Dembner Books

Published by Red Dembner Enterprises Corp.,
80 Eighth Avenue,
New York, N.Y. 10011

Distributed by W. W. Norton & Company, Inc.,
500 Fifth Avenue,
New York, N.Y. 10110

Copyright © 1982, 1989 by Jerome Z. Litt, M.D.

Revised, expanded, and updated edition.

Library of Congress Cataloging-in-Publication Data

Litt, Jerome Z.
  Your skin: from acne to zits / Jerome Z. Litt.
    p.   cm.
  Includes index.
  ISBN 0-942637-13-5 : $9.95
  1. Skin—Care and hygiene.   I. Title.
RL87.L57   1989
616.5—dc19   89-30965
                                                  CIP

Designed by Antler & Baldwin, Inc.

Second Printing, 1989

CONTENTS

To Vel, my best reward.

INTRODUCTION

The skin.

Not "skin." *The* skin. The house we live in.

What is this bag we call the skin—this fantastic envelope that possesses some of the most extraordinary mechanisms in the entire body? It is an organ of the body—a marvelously efficient apparatus that nourishes, guards, and protects us twenty-four hours a day.

When laid out flat, the skin of an average adult would measure some twenty square feet; it would weigh about nine pounds. That's a lot of organ—one of the largest and heaviest of the body. Also the most abused and maligned organ of the body.

Considering those "thousand natural shocks that skin is heir to," its continuing function and lack of complaint is nothing short of amazing.

How do we treat this remarkable mechanism? We dig and rub and scratch it. We expose it to all the elements—extremes of heat and cold, sun, wind, rain, and snow. We cut it, shave it, pick it, squeeze it, pinch it, and twist it. We scrub it, pull it, and bend it. We rub it, slap it, punch it, and knead it.

In the name of Beauty, we paint it and mark it and spray it. In the name of Health, we massage it and scorch it in the steam room and sauna. Name another organ that can stand up to all that! Yet it survives!

We never think of our skin as we do our heart, liver, lungs, kidneys, brain, or any other "important" organ. To many of us, this complex body stocking we wear so casually is just a sac to hold our insides in, a bag containing some watery stuff and bones. But the skin is an important, vital, viable, living mechanism without which the human organism cannot survive.

Think of what your skin, the most visible of all bodily organs and the only body tissue that is exposed to dry air, does to serve you:

- With its fifteen feet of blood vessels per square inch, your skin helps to regulate your body temperature, making it possible for you to adjust to extremes of cold and heat.
- The large integument that covers your body—what we call skin—represents the first line of defense against harmful germs that constantly try to break through and invade your tissues.
- Despite its soft and elastic appearance, your skin is tough enough to withstand a variety of shocks and blows, acting as a cushion to protect your deeper, more vital organs from harm.
- This porous yet leakproof organ is a protective barrier between your internal body systems and the hostile environment, preventing poisonous chemicals from penetrating your deeper tissues. At the same time, it prevents the outward loss of water, blood, minerals, hormones, and other essential body fluids. A genuine waterproof sac!
- Recent advances in dermatologic research have shown that your skin helps to metabolize and detoxify certain drugs and potentially dangerous environmental chemicals. If a harmful substance lands on the skin and begins to penetrate, various enzymes in the skin will break it down into harmless constituents.
- Skin cells produce substances—interferons and interleukins—known to be important to the immune defense system.
- The skin is your largest organ of sensation, allowing you to perceive heat and cold and various tactile impressions, such as pain. It is the principal organ of communication between you and your environment—the "switchboard" that receives

and transmits such information as "the stove is hot," "that knife is sharp," "this pillow is soft."
- It is an organ of excretion, a vast garbage disposal system continually eliminating body wastes through more than two million sweat pores.
- Your skin protects you against the harmful effects of the sun's rays by absorbing them and converting them into dark pigment (tan) to prevent further damage.
- Your skin is supplied with oil glands—100 per square inch—which secrete sebum, the oily material responsible for maintaining the resiliency and elasticity of the skin surface.
- The skin acts as a storage house for water as well as for various nutriments, such as sugar and calcium.
- It helps in the production of vitamin D (which is really a hormone). This controls the absorption of calcium and phosphorus—minerals vital for the development of strong bones and for the prevention of rickets.
- Your skin is a mirror of what occurs below the surface—a warning signal of systemic diseases, such as diabetes, shingles, leukemia, and cancer, which often manifest themselves as skin problems long before there is positive evidence of these internal conditions.
- Finally, your "decorative wrapping" is endowed with a special capacity to reflect human passions and sentiment. As a mirror of emotions the skin is without peer. Livid with rage, pale with fright, blushing with shame. The sweating palm, the anxious pallor. All are release mechanisms of the skin that express combinations of inner feelings and skin reactions to tension, anxiety, and stress.

This, then, is your skin—"the envelope that encloses the letter of your biologic destiny" —that remarkable apparatus that spends a lifetime helping you adjust to your environment.

But we are not kind to our skin. We abuse it. And although we spend $20 billion a year on skin care and cosmetics, we do not understand it. Only when the itching or burning or pain become unbearable or when the cosmetic disfigurement becomes embarrassing do we begin to take it seriously.

While the skin is strong and tough, it is also delicate and fragile. The cure-all in a jar that promises relief from such diverse conditions as acne, warts, eczema, dry skin, poison ivy dermatitis, genital herpes, and psoriasis is deceptive and misleading. One salve or lotion cannot be useful for a dozen different ailments, just as Cinderella's slipper will not fit every foot.

There are over one thousand different diseases and conditions that can affect the skin, hair, and nails. Everyone will, at one time or another, develop some type of problem that deals with this large integumentary system.

Warts, dandruff, dry skin, moles, athlete's foot. Excess hair or not enough hair. Rashes from the sun, from germs, from poison ivy. Insect bites, cold sores, hives, rectal itch. Large pores, wrinkles, stretch marks or scars.

Job had boils.

Caesar was bald. Queen Elizabeth I lost every hair on her body.

Napoleon had scabies.

Tolstoy had canker sores. Wagner had eczema.

Ernest Hemingway had psoriasis.

Winston Churchill had a persistent, intolerable, dry skin itch.

Dr. Tom Dooley had a melanoma and died from it.

Lyndon B. Johnson had skin cancer. So did Ronald and Nancy Reagan.

Soviet leader, Mikhail S. Gorbachev has a large birthmark on his scalp.

Golda Meir, Arthur Rubinstein, and Richard Nixon suffered from severe shingles.

Telly Savalas has a mole. So does Elizabeth Taylor and Madonna.

Tens of millions of people all over the world have acne, warts, and eczema.

Your male friends may have hair loss, athlete's foot, or jock itch; your female friends may complain of large pores, stretch marks, and "zits." And almost all adult women have cellulite!

Your children will have impetigo, diaper rash, ringworm, acne, warts, cradle cap, birthmarks, and insect bites.

Your parents will develop dry skin, wrinkles, skin tumors, leg ulcers, and shingles.

And how many of you are plagued with canker sores? Rectal itch? What about the eight million Americans who have psoriasis? And the countless millions who are frustrated by eczema?

No one can escape.

WHAT THIS BOOK CAN DO FOR YOU

In the following pages you'll learn about a few dozen conditions that commonly affect the skin, hair, and nails. Many of them are not diseases in the sense that they cause some bodily dysfunction, but they are important enough to affect your general well-being and psychological health. You'll learn something about the causes and symptoms of these disorders and the different methods doctors use to treat them.

At the end of many of the chapters, you'll find sections describing what you yourself can do to prevent, manage, or eliminate particular skin, hair, and nail conditions. Please understand there is no magic in the treatment of skin disease. The skin, like every other organ, can develop "instant" maladies—maladies that may take weeks or months to heal or improve. The sunburn that develops in an hour, the cold sores or poison ivy dermatitis that can begin overnight, the zits or boils that erupt in a day, the hives that appear in minutes from aspirin or penicillin—all may take days or weeks of constant medication to get them under control.

The products that I mention in these treatment sections are "over-the-counter" medications which you can purchase at your local drugstore without a doctor's prescription. A few of these are oral medications, medications that you take by mouth. Others are "topical," or surface, medications that you apply directly on the area you are treating.

When using any medication, follow the directions on the label or the directions that I have provided. Be careful to note any special precautions. You must realize that all people do not respond alike to every medication—local, oral, or by injection. The salve that's so beneficial for Portia might cause Stevie to break out. The soothing lotion for Jacob might cause burning on Elizabeth's skin. And there are some people who, unfortunately, develop an allergy (sensitivity) to almost every variety of surface medication.

If you find that a preparation causes some unpleasant symptom, such as burning, stinging, pain, or increased itching, discontinue it at once. It could be that you are—or have become—allergic to one or more of the ingredients in it. If this occurs, try a different type or brand of medication.

While I have mentioned scores of products for the management of dozens of skin, hair, and nail disorders, there are literally hundreds of others that may serve the same purposes. The products I have listed are ones that I personally prescribe and recommend in my private practice of dermatology—a practice that numbers well over 90,000 patients. I have tested these products over the years, and while I cannot speak for *all* the other 7,500 dermatologists in this country, a majority of them recommend the same preparations.

Most importantly, do not hesitate to see your dermatologist. This book does not replace his or her expertise. Rather, it aims to help you better understand your skin and how to live in it.

WHERE GOOD SKIN BEGINS

What does good skin look and feel like? Does the face or body of a fashion model or entertainment star pop into your head? Actually, glamour has nothing to do with it. You can't tell good skin by magazine photos or movie close-ups since photographers and make-up artists are trained to trick the eye.

Underneath it all, healthy skin is smooth, soft, elastic, fresh, and clear of blemishes. If that's not what you see when you look in a mirror, there may be a lot of reasons why not.

The way your skin looks and feels, its condition and health, depend on the following factors, some of which you can't control:

- Your heredity
- Your age
- Your general health
- Medications you may be taking
- Your diet (you are what you eat!)
- Exercise and rest
- How you take care of your skin
- The amount of sun exposure you've had
- Whether you're male or female.

7

HEREDITY
Heredity plays a big part in what your skin is and what it will be. If you are black, your skin is stronger than that of your white friends. Black skin is thicker and tougher, has greater protection from the sun's dangerous rays, and wrinkles much less—and much later—than fair skin.

Black people, even when they're seventy or eighty years old, usually have fewer wrinkles than white people who are in their fifties. And, if a black person hasn't been in the sun a lot during his or her lifetime, you may *never* see a wrinkle.

If you are blue-eyed, blonde, and fair-skinned with Scandinavian or Irish relatives, your skin will usually be thin and delicate. This type of skin can't take exposure to the sun, wind, cold, or other harsh weather. It also develops wrinkles sooner than darker skin does.

AGE
We're all getting older every day, but our skin ages differently, depending on heredity, general health, and how you have taken care of your skin. There are, however, some general stages in our skin's life.

Young people's skins are more delicate and thinner than those of adults. Infants with diaper rash and young children who are covered with scrapes, scratches, and bruises have less protection from the outside world than the adult whose skin has become toughened to handle the nicks and bumps of everyday living. The teenager whose oil-producing glands are increasing their activity will develop oily skin, oily hair, and acne.

When you get old, your skin becomes very thin and fragile, just as it was when you were a baby. Bumping your skin even a little bit can cause large bruises and blemishes. As your skin ages, it becomes saggy. Changes in hormones cut down the skin's oil supply and the skin becomes rough and dry, and "age spots" develop.

GENERAL HEALTH
Your skin actually mirrors what's going on inside your body. So to have healthy skin, you must be in good physical and emotional health.

Many diseases, infections, and illnesses show up on the skin in several ways. For example, diabetes can cause dry skin, itching, pigment and nail changes, and yeast infections. Hepatitis and other liver disorders may create terrible itching or hives. Gall bladder trouble and some blood disorders will cause your skin to turn yellow. Hormone imbalances can change your skin color or make you lose your hair. Or cause you to grow too much hair. Certain blood diseases can cause itching, hives, and shingles, while lack of vitamins can bring on cracked lips, hair loss, dry skin, and mouth ulcers.

Stress, worry, and other emotional problems can show up as changes in your skin, such as acne pimples, hair loss, or differences in your skin's color, texture, or elasticity.

MEDICATIONS

Taking vitamins, diet pills, and many other medications can change the appearance of your skin, hair, and nails. Very dry skin can result from taking thyroid medication and high doses of vitamin A.

Hives can develop from hundreds of medications, usually aspirin, penicillin, and sulfa. Acne and oily skin are frequent side effects of low-dose birth control pills, anti-epilepsy medication, and cortisone-like drugs. You can develop sun poisoning if you get too much sun while taking sulfa drugs, high blood pressure pills, oral contraceptives, or medicines with tetracycline. A rash that looks a lot like measles can show up if you're taking penicillin, ampicillin, sleeping pills, or Librium. Low-dose birth control pills, thyroid medication, male hormones, and a variety of drugs used to treat cancer, can all cause hair to fall out.

All of these side effects shouldn't discourage you from taking your medicines, but you should know what *might* happen when you do. If you think you are developing an unusual reaction from some type of medication, check with the doctor who prescribed it.

DIET

Since the living cells that produce your skin, hair, and nails depend on what you eat for their supply of nutrients, it is important that you feed your body well. In other words, "eat a well-balanced diet."

Poor eating habits can cause temporary hair loss, cracks in the corners of your mouth, and changes in your nails. Your skin may bruise easily, heal slowly, and look dull, drab, and "ashy." A good diet keeps your skin healthy, helps your skin have good tone, texture, and color, and protects your skin from disease. You shouldn't have to take vitamin supplements if you eat right. There is no proof that swallowing extra vitamins or minerals does anything good for your skin.

Rashes and other problems can occur when you eat certain foods. If you're allergic to penicillin, some cheeses (such as Roquefort and blue) can cause hives. If you like seaweed salad, you should know that kelp can cause zits. Eating too many carrots, oranges, or tomatoes can turn your skin yellow. Quinine (in quinine water) can cause bruises and hives. Seafood, chocolate, strawberries, and many other foods can bring on bouts of cold sores on the lips.

EXERCISE AND REST

Regular exercise is an important part of staying healthy. It takes care of boredom, tension, and anxiety, keeps your body in good shape, and enhances the color and texture of your skin. Exercising improves the circulation of the blood which then provides nourishment to the skin to build new cells, helps the skin get rid of impurities, and keeps it looking healthy and glowing.

When you don't get enough rest, circulation is cut down and the skin receives less oxygen and nourishment. As a result, your skin may look dull and sallow, acne zits can flare up, and dark circles can appear under your eyes. Suggestion: get your beauty sleep.

HOW YOU TAKE CARE OF YOUR SKIN

The NUMBER ONE rule for having good, clear skin is to clean it the right way. A clean skin is a healthy skin.

Proper cleansing removes the irritating and poisonous agents and germs that could hurt your skin or, by absorption through the skin, actually cause harm to other parts of your body. There are many ways to clean your skin, but the good, old-fashioned soap and water routine is really the best, most efficient, and least expensive method.

What are some of the things you want to wash away to keep your skin clean and healthy-looking?

First of all, you have substances produced by your own body:

- Dead, horny cells from the very upper layers of the skin. If these are not regularly washed off, your complexion will be dull and lifeless.

- Sweat from the millions of sweat glands all over your body. A lot of this sweat is responsible for body odor.
- Sebum, the oily material that gives the skin its softness and elasticity. When this oily substance builds up, acne pimples result.
- Ear wax and old hair and nail cells, just sitting there on your skin, up to no good.

Then there are the substances coming from the environment:

- Pollutants found in the air, such as smoke, soot, dust, pollens, and exhaust fumes from cars, busses, trucks.
- Materials around your work place, such as grease and grime from gas stations and fast-food restaurants.
- Things found in your own home. These could be paints, glues, resins, clothing, bedding, carpeting, house sprays— even belly-button lint!
- All the bottles, jars, and sprays of "who-knows-what" you apply to your skin by design, such as cosmetics, suntan lotions, perfumes, and surface medications.
- Various "friendly" germs which live normally on your skin.

Regular washing with soap and water rinses and flushes this skin garbage away, cleans the pores, reduces odor, and cuts down the risk of infection and disease. Your clean skin will look soft, glowing, and healthy. Its circulation will improve, encouraging the growth of healthy cells, and your skin will breathe better. All this, by just washing your face three times a day.

A word on cleansing creams used mostly to remove make-up. While your make-up seems to disappear, you're actually left with an irritating combination of cream, leftover make-up, and other impurities that were already on the skin. This leftover mess not only irritates your skin but also can clog the pores, leading to blackheads and whiteheads. If you try to remove it with tissues, you only further clog up the pore openings.

Let's face it, only soap and water will really get your skin clean. Washing your face three times a day with a mild, gentle soap is the most important advice I can give. If you want to take off make-up with a cleansing cream, follow it up with soap and water to get rid of all that mess than can only cause problems.

The kind of soap you use on your face is a matter of personal choice, but watch out for the ones that are irritating or can't be completely rinsed off. The so-called cold cream soaps, although they are fairly mild and gentle, always leave a film of cold cream, plugging up the oil glands which are already working hard to get rid of their normal oil supply. The deodorant and antibacterial soaps can be especially irritating to facial skin because they leave a residue of chemicals on your skin to destroy germs. If you have a body odor problem, use these types of soaps only below the neck.

Do your face a favor and use a mild, gentle soap that does its cleansing job well, rinses off easily, and leaves nothing behind. Try any of the following:

Cetaphil Lotion (Owen/Allercreme)

Lowila Cake (Westwood)

Purpose Soap (Johnson & Johnson)

THE AMOUNT OF SUN EXPOSURE YOU'VE HAD

To keep your skin healthy, you must learn to protect it. And the most harmful agent you must protect it from is the sun. Damaging sun rays can cause wrinkles and skin cancer as well. They're really hard on people with light hair, blue eyes, and fair skin.

A golden, bronzed body is beautiful! We think it's healthy and desirable. But a tan is nothing more than your body's marvelous defense against the dangerous effects of the sun's harmful rays, the ones that lead to early aging of the skin, wrinkles and ultimately, skin cancer.

You absolutely cannot tan without damaging your skin. Sun damage is cumulative and irreversible. Your skin is like a sponge and a bank: it soaks up all those rays and stores them. Forever!

The best protection from the sun is to avoid it completely. Second best is to apply a good sunscreen with a Sun Protection Factor of at least 15. (See page 157 for recommendations.)

FEMALE OR MALE

Finally, the health of your skin, its color, texture, and strength will depend on your sex.

The next time you're at the shopping mall or in a crowd, take a look at white couples in their fifties or sixties. If the man and woman are about the same age, you'll probably notice that the woman looks about ten years older than the man. Her facial skin will appear drier and less elastic, and she'll have more wrinkles. Why? Several reasons:

- Because of the male hormone (androgen), a man's dermis (the lower layer of the skin) is thicker than a woman's. As a result of this extra thickness, he is better protected from the weather, such as cold and wind, and less likely to have aging damage from the sun.

- Women's thinner skin also may be damaged more by outside influences such as cosmetics, facial exercises, and massages.
- Men's collagen fibers (the fibers in the dermis, the lower layer of the skin, that give the skin its strength and elasticity) are more tightly packed together. That's why men don't have droopy skin around the throat or little vertical lines on the upper lip, both problems for older women.
- In addition, the same hormones that make men's skin thicker make it oilier than women's, giving it a more elastic and flexible look and feel.

If you understand all of these conditions that affect the health of your skin—and what you can and can't do about them—you'll be on the right road to taking care of that marvelous organ we call skin. And you really should. It has to last you a lifetime.

SKIN CONDITIONS FROM THE TOP DOWN AN ANATOMICAL GUIDE

What's this rash? Why does it itch? What do I have?

Let's say you have a rash on your elbows. It looks peculiar, but it doesn't itch. What could it be? Should you be worried?

Instead of going through the entire book looking up each condition or disorder, you can use this section to go straight to the chapter about that particular part of your body.

For example: You just developed this non-itchy rash on your elbows. Look under the section on "arms and forearms" on page 23 and find out what type of non-itchy disorder might develop on your elbows. Could it be psoriasis?

This section is arranged in order "from the top." While this simplified anatomical guide can't cover every rash, growth, or variation, it can give you some idea of what you MAY have and what you probably do NOT have.

Rashes and growths can occur on virtually every portion of your skin and mucous membranes. The following list includes the most common problems that affect these portions of the body. Some of these disorders are not covered in this book, so please check with your dermatologist if you're concerned about a particular condition.

SCALP
 RASHES
  1. **Dandruff:** Scaling, flaking, and itching. [*See page 101*]
  2. **Seborrheic Dermatitis:** Scaling, itching, redness, accompanied by a red, scaly rash on the sides of the nose and eyebrows. [*See page 102*]
  3. **Psoriasis:** Thick, scaly crusts and patches. May or may not itch. May have similar red or silvery-scaly patches on knees and elbows. [*See page 54*]
  4. **Eczema:** Red, weeping, itchy, crusted areas. May have itchy rash in bends of elbows and behind knees. [*See page 49*]
  5. **Head Lice:** Intensely itchy rash, mainly on back of head. Look for nits as well as friends or relatives with same condition. [*See page 75*]
  6. **Allergy Rashes:** Red, weeping, itchy areas. Have you been using anything new? Hair dye, shampoos, hair tonic, hair pins, bobby pins, curlers? Any rash on the neck? [*See page 84*]
  7. **Shingles:** Itchy, painful rash with water blisters. May involve the forehead, ear, and neck. Affects one side of the head only. [*See page 67*]
  RECOMMENDATION: See your dermatologist.
  8. **Lupus Erythematosus:** Complete loss of hair in a shiny, scarred, pink or white patch. No itching. [*See page 181*]
  RECOMMENDATION: See your dermatologist.
  9. **Pyoderma:** An impetigo-like infection accompanied by weeping, oozing, and painful crusts. May be accompanied by fever and big "knots" behind the ears. [*See Impetigo, page 70*]
  RECOMMENDATION: See your dermatologist.

 TUMORS
  1. **Warts:** Grayish growths of varying size. Occasionally bleed when injured by combs and brushes. Warts may appear on the face and neck as well. [*See page 46*]
  2. **Moles:** Flesh-colored growths of varying size. May be smooth or pebbly. May or may not have hair growing in them. [*See page 201*]
  RECOMMENDATION: See your dermatologist if you notice any change in a mole.
  3. **Wens (sebaceous cysts):** Smooth, round, dome-like, soft or moderately hard tumors filled with greasy, cheese-like, odoriferous material.
  RECOMMENDATION: See your dermatologist

MISCELLANEOUS

1. **Alopecia areata:** Loss of hair in coin-shaped patches. Areas are smooth and completely hairless. [*See page 110*]

RECOMMENDATION: See your dermatologist.

FOREHEAD

RASHES

1. **Acne:** Pimples and pustules, often appearing elsewhere on the face as well. [*See page 39*]

2. **Seborrheic Dermatitis:** Redness, scaling, and itching near the hairline, often accompanied by heavy dandruff. [*See page 102*]

3. **Eczema:** Scaling, itching, and redness. May have itchy rash in bends of elbows and knees. [*See page 49*]

4. **Allergy Rashes:** Redness, itching, and occasionally, small water blisters. Have you been exposed to poison ivy? Anything new in the way of hats, headbands, hair nets, bathing caps, hair dyes, permanents, or cosmetics? [*page 84*]

5. **Shingles:** Painful and itchy blisters located on one side and extending around to the ear, upper eyelid, and side of scalp on that side only. [*See page 67*]

RECOMMENDATION: See your dermatologist.

6. **Psoriasis:** Redness and silvery scales extending down from hairline. Usually no itching. May have similar patches on knees and elbows. [*See page 54*]

7. **Rosacea:** Red pimples and pustules accompanied by a similar rash over the cheeks and nose. [*See page 188*]

TUMORS

1. **Moles:** Often brown or flesh-colored. [*See page 201*]

RECOMMENDATION: See your dermatologist for any change in size, color, or texture of a mole.

2. **Warts:** Grayish lesions of varying size. May be single or multiple. May be clusters of flat warts which are slightly elevated and smooth. [*See page 46*]

EYELIDS

RASHES

Because the skin of the eyelids is thin and exposed, it is among the most commonly affected parts of the body when it comes to skin disorders. Swollen eyelids are particularly common. The swelling is more severe when you first awaken in the morning.

1. **Allergy rashes:** Redness, itching, swelling in the morning. Scaly, dark, and thickened when chronic. More common on the upper eyelids. [*See page 84*]

2. **Hives:** Itching, stinging, and burning welts accompanied by hives elsewhere. [*See page 79*]

3. **Seborrheic Dermatitis:** Greasy, scaly, red patches. Often associated with severe dandruff and seborrheic dermatitis behind the ears, and on the sides of nose. The eyelids margins (edges) may have stuck-on crusts. [*See page 102*]

4. **Eczema:** Red, itchy, scaly patches. May also appear in bends of elbows and knees. [*See page 49*]

5. **Lice infestation:** Small, white nits (eggs) stuck on to the hairs at the margin of the eyelid. Look for lice elsewhere. [*See page 75*]

6. **Rosacea:** The margins of the eyelids may be red with small pus pimples. Accompanied by redness, pimples, and pustules on the cheeks and nose. [*See page 188*]

TUMORS

1. **Whiteheads:** Small, shiny, firm, translucent or yellow, pin-head-sized cysts. Have you been using a greasy or oily makeup? A greasy moisturizer? [*See page 40*]

2. **Dimple Warts** (Molluscum Contagiosum): Pin-head to match-head sized, single or multiple, smooth nodules, often with a central depression (like a bellybutton). [*See page 168*]

RECOMMENDATION: See your dermatologist since they are contagious.

NOSE

RASHES

1. **Acne:** Oiliness, blackheads, pimples and pustules. Will probably show up elsewhere on face, as well. [*See page 39*]

2. **Seborrheic Dermatitis:** Red, greasy scales in the folds and along the sides of the nose. Usually no itching. Often associated with dandruff and seborrheic dermatitis elsewhere. [*See page 102*]

3. **Allergy Rashes:** Red, itchy, scaly areas. May be due to nickel or rubber in bridge of eyeglasses or colored facial tissues. [*See page 84*]

4. **Impetigo:** Honey-colored crusts, usually over the nostrils and lower portion of the nose. Check to see if any relatives or friends have a similar condition. [*See page 70*]

5. **Lupus Erythematosus (LE):** Pink or depigmented scarred patches associated with LE elsewhere (cheeks, scalp, chin). [*See page 181*]

RECOMMENDATION: See your dermatologist.

6. **Cold Sores (herpes simplex):** Small, itchy blisters on a reddened base. May recur in the same place again and again. [*See page 61*]

7. **Shingles:** Painful and itchy blisters over nose tip. May mean involvement of the eye, which can be serious. Look for shingles on the forehead and in the scalp. [*See page 67*]

RECOMMENDATION: See your dermatologist

8. **Frostbite:** Tingling, burning, pain, and, occasionally, numbness over the tip of the nose. Due to exposure to frigid temperatures and inadequate protection of nose. [*See page 169*]

RECOMMENDATION: See your dermatologist.

9. **Rosacea:** Redness with pimples and pustules accompanied by a similar rash over the cheeks and forehead. In long-standing cases, this might progress to rhinophyma—a W.C. Fields' nose. [*See page 188*]

CHEEKS
RASHES
1. **Acne:** Oiliness, blackheads, pimples and pustules. [*See page 39*]

2. **Impetigo:** Honey-colored, stuck-on crusts. Occasionally itchy. Look for impetigo elsewhere (nose, lips). [*See page 70*]

3. **Allergy Rashes:** Redness, swelling, itching, scaling. May be tiny blisters. Have you been using any new cosmetics, soaps, acne medications, hair dyes? Exposure to poison ivy? Any fumes (paints or sprays)? [*See page 84*]

4. **Eczema:** Itchy, scaly, thickening of the skin. Look for similar condition in bends of elbows and knees. [*See page 49*]

5. **Cold Sores (herpes simplex):** Small, itchy blisters on a reddened base. May recur in the same place. Look for cold sores elsewhere. [*See page 61*]

6. **Lupus Erythematosus:** Sharply-demarcated, pink or whitish, scarred patches. No itching. May have similar patches over nose and scalp. [*See page 181*]

RECOMMENDATION: See your dermatologist.

7. **Rosacea:** Red, pimply eruption accompanied by a similar condition over the nose and forehead. [*See page 188*]

TUMORS

1. **Moles:** Flesh-colored to brownish, flat or raised, hairy or hairless lesions of varying size. [*See page 201*]

RECOMMENDATION: For any change in a mole, see your dermatologist.

2. **Warts:** Single or multiple grayish lesions of varying size. Flat warts are smooth, slightly-raised, soft, flesh-colored to tan lesions. They are often numerous and appear on the forehead as well. [*See page 46*]

MISCELLANEOUS

1. **Alopecia areata:** Patchy hair loss in men's bearded area. Look for alopecia areata in scalp and eyelashes. [*See page 110*]

LIPS

RASHES

1. **Allergy Rashes:** Redness, scaling, and itching; occasional, small water blisters. Any new lipstick or other lip cosmetics? New toothpaste or mouth wash? Gum? Foods? [*See page 84*]

2. **Cold Sores (herpes simplex):** Small, itchy water blisters. Very common on upper lip. Does it recur? Can you track it down to a certain food? [*See page 61*]

3. **Hives:** Swelling of the lips with itching. Can be very severe (called "bull hives"). Look for hives elsewhere. Probably due to some food (seafood or nuts or chocolate) or medication (aspirin or penicillin tablets). [*See page 79*]

4. **Perleche:** Cracks at the corners of the mouth. May be due to appliances in the mouth (braces, retainers, dentures) or gum-chewing.

RECOMMENDATION: Keep mouth dry at all times, discontinue chewing gum, and do not eat raw fruit (except when cut up in small pieces). See your dermatologist if it does not clear up after a few days.

5. **Canker Sores:** Painful ulcerations accompanied by similar lesions inside the mouth. [*See page 162*]

TUMORS

1. **Warts:** Grayish-looking lesions; single or multiple. Usually seen over the lower lip. [*See page 46*]

2. **Whiteheads:** Small, yellowish, shiny lesions around the lip margins, caused most often by greasy lip cosmetics. [*See page 40*]

CHIN
RASHES
1. **Acne:** Blackheads, pimples, and pustules with some oiliness. Often there are acne lesions elsewhere on the face. [*See page 39*]
2. **Impetigo:** Honey-colored, stuck-on crusts, with or without itching. Look for impetigo elsewhere (nose, cheeks) and relatives or friends with the same condition. [*See page 70*]
3. **Allergy rashes:** Redness, itching, scaling, and occasional blisters. Have you been using any new cosmetics or soaps? Shaving preparations? Any new topical medications? Bubble gum? Kissing someone with a heavy beard? [*See page 84*]
4. **Lupus Erythematosus:** White or pinkish, round patches with well-defined borders. No itching. May have similar patches elsewhere on face. [*See page 181*]
RECOMMENDATION: See your dermatologist.
5. **Rosacea:** Redness and pimples accompanied by a similar eruption over the cheeks and nose. [*See page 188*]

TUMORS
1. **Warts:** Single or multiple grayish lesions of varying size. Can be flat or smooth. Look for warts elsewhere on face. [*See page 46*]
2. **Moles:** Tan or brown, hairy or hairless lesions of varying size. [*See page 201*]

EARS
RASHES
1. **Seborrheic Dermatitis:** Scaling, redness, and itching particularly behind the ears. May be accompanied by red, scaly rash on sides of nose and severe dandruff. [*See page 102*]
2. **Allergy Rashes:** Redness, itching, and occasional small water blisters. May be due to metal or chemical in eyeglass temples, earrings, hearing aids, ear drops, nail polish, cosmetics, hair dyes, shampoos, hair sprays, scalp lotions, etc. [*See page 84*]
3. **Psoriasis:** Thick, silvery-white, scaly patches. May have similar patches on elbows, knees, and scalp. [*See page 54*]
4. **Eczema:** Red, weeping, itchy, and sometimes crusted areas in and behind ears. Itchy rash may also appear in bends of elbows and behind knees. [*See page 49*]

5. **Impetigo:** Honey-colored crusted areas. May have similar crusted areas over nostrils and around mouth. [*See page 70*]

6. **Shingles:** Itchy, painful rash with blisters over one ear with similar areas over the neck and scalp on the same side. [*See page 67*]

RECOMMENDATION: See your dermatologist.

7. **Frostbite:** Tingling, burning, pain, and, occasionally, numbness over the rim and lobes of the ears. Due to exposure to frigid temperatures and inadequate protection of ears. [*See page 169*]

TUMORS

1. **Moles:** Flesh-colored or tan, hairy or hairless growths. [*See page 201*]

RECOMMENDATION: For any change in a mole, see your dermatologist.

2. **Warts:** Grayish growths of varying size. May be solitary or multiple. [*See page 46*]

3. **Cysts:** Small, hard, movable growths usually in ear lobes. Occurs often after ear-piercing and represents a plugging up of small oil glands in the earlobe.

RECOMMENDATION: See your dermatologist.

4. **Keratoses:** Scaly, crusted, wart-like growths of varying size over the rim of the ears. [*See page 203*]

RECOMMENDATION: See your dermatologist, as these may be premalignant lesions.

NECK

RASHES

1. **Allergy Rashes:** Redness, itching, occasional small water blisters. May be due to chemicals in nail polish, cosmetics, hair dyes and lotions, perfumes, furs, dyed clothing, soap, or some type of surface medication. [*See page 84*]

2. **Impetigo:** Honey-colored crusts. May be accompanied by similar rash on nostrils, cheeks, and elsewhere. [*See page 70*]

3. **Seborrheic Dermatitis:** Scaling, itching, and redness. May have a similar rash on sides of nose. [*See page 102*]

4. **Eczema:** Red, weeping, and itching areas. May have a similar, itchy rash in the bends of the elbows and behind the knees. [*See page 49*]

5. **Pityriasis Rosea:** Pale rose, oval patches, usually not itchy.

Shows up as a "herald" patch followed by Christmas tree-like pattern. [*See page 82*]

6. **Shingles:** Itchy, painful rash with small water blisters on one side of the neck. May affect the ear and cheek on the same side. [*See page 67*]

RECOMMENDATION: See your dermatologist.

7. **Ringworm:** A well-demarcated, round or oval, itchy, scaly patch with a red border and a clear center. Check if you've been exposed to an animal (usually a puppy or kitten) or a person with ringworm.

RECOMMENDATION: See your dermatologist.

8. **Folliculitis:** Inflammation of hair follicles, commonly occurring in black men (pseudofolliculitis barbae). Also known as "razor bumps." [*See page 36*]

9. **Acne:** Pimples and pustules, and occasional cysts and scars over the back of the neck. Very common in young men. Scarred areas over the back of the neck in black men are known as acne keloid. May be accompanied by acne lesions elsewhere. [*See page 39*]

10. **Ichthyosis:** Dry, grayish, thickened and scaly areas accompanied by a similar rash over the trunk or extremities. [*See page 177*]

TUMORS

1. **Warts:** Grayish or flesh-colored growths of varying size. May be single or multiple. Very difficult to eradicate in men who shave. [*See page 46*]

2. **Dimple Warts:** Small, pearly nodules, each with a central depression or bellybutton. Common in wrestlers. [*See page 168*]

RECOMMENDATION: Since they are contagious, see your dermatologist.

ARMPITS

Armpits, because of their hair and sweat glands and the considerable amount of friction they get, are especially troubled by irritation, inflammation, and infection.

RASHES

1. **Allergy Rashes:** Redness, itching, and on occasion, small water blisters. May be due to antiperspirants and deodorants, hair removers, cosmetics, clothing dyes, dress shields, and strong soaps. Shaving aggravates these rashes. [*See page 84*]

2. **Seborrheic Dermatitis:** Scaling, itching, and redness. May be accompanied by excess dandruff and scaling and redness on the sides of the nose and scalp. [*See page 102*]

3. **Scabies:** Intense itching, particularly at night. May also have itching over wrists, fingerwebs, and genitals. [*See page 77*]

4. **Lice:** Intense itching along with itching in the pubic area and groins. Look for small eggs (nits) glued to the hair and close friends who have a similar itch. [*See page 75*]

5. **Boil:** A painful and tender swelling in the dome of the armpit due to infection by certain bacteria.
RECOMMENDATION: See your dermatologist.

6. **Ringworm:** A well-demarcated, itchy, round or oval patch with a red border and clear center. Check if you've been exposed to a person or animal (usually a puppy or kitten) with ringworm.
RECOMMENDATION: See your dermatologist.

7. **Shingles:** Itchy, painful rash with small water blisters in only one armpit. May have a similar rash over the shoulder and arm on the same side. [*See page 67*]
RECOMMENDATION: See your dermatologist.

TUMORS

1. **Dimple Warts:** Small, pearly nodules with a central depression or bellybutton. Often seen in wrestlers. [*See page 168*]
RECOMMENDATION: Since these are contagious, see your dermatologist.

2. **Skin Tags:** Small, fleshy growths that are very common in the armpits and are usually hereditary. They are "friendly" tumors and never become malignant.

ARMS AND FOREARMS
RASHES

1. **Allergy Rashes:** Redness, itching, and occasional small water blisters. May be due to a variety of chemicals, including plants (poison ivy), dyes in clothing, soaps, detergents, cosmetics, and work-related substances. [*See page 84*]

2. **Eczema:** Red, weeping, itchy rash, particularly in the bends of the elbows. [*See page 49*]

3. **Acne:** Pimples and pustules over the upper arms. May have acne on face, chest, back, and elsewhere. [*See page 39*]

4. **Shingles:** An itchy, painful rash with small blisters over one arm and forearm. May have a similar rash over the shoulder and neck on the same side. [*See page 67*]
RECOMMENDATION: See your dermatologist.

5. **Ringworm:** A well-demarcated, itchy, round or oval patch with a red border and clear center. Check to see if you've been exposed to a person or animal (puppy or kitten) with ringworm.
RECOMMENDATION: See your dermatologist.

6. **Keratosis Pilaris:** A very common rash over the backs of the arms that looks and feels like a cheese grater. This is a harmless condition that often disappears by itself after a number of years. Improves in the summertime.

7. **Ichthyosis:** Dry, scaly, fishskin-like eruption accompanied by a similar rash over the legs and trunk. [*See page 177*]

ELBOWS
Comparatively few conditions affect the elbow areas.
RASHES
1. **Psoriasis:** Thick, silvery-white, scaly patches. Seldom itches. The elbows, along with the knees, are the most common locations for psoriasis. Patches often seen in the scalp as well. [*See page 54*]

2. **Scabies:** Intense itching, particularly at night. May be accompanied by itching over the wrists, fingerwebs, and genitals. [*See page 77*]
RECOMMENDATION: See your dermatologist.

3. **Allergy Rashes:** Redness and itching in a well-demarcated patch. May be due to a new article of clothing, leaning elbows on a freshly-painted or waxed table top, or fabric softeners used in the dryer. [*See page 84*]

TUMORS
1. **Warts:** Grayish or flesh-colored growths. May be single or in groups. Often resistant to all forms of treatment. [*See page 46*]

WRISTS
RASHES
1. **Lichen Planus:** Itchy, violet-colored, slightly-raised "bumps" over the inner wrists. May have a similar rash on the ankles and small of the back. [*See page 179*]

2. **Scabies:** Intense itching, particularly at night. May have similar itching between the fingers and in genital area. [*See page 77*]
RECOMMENDATION: See your dermatologist.

3. **Allergy Rashes:** Redness and itching with occasional, small water blisters. May be due to contact with watches, watchbands, or bracelets. [*page 84*]

4. **Ringworm:** Round or oval, scaly patch with a sharp red border and clear center. Check for exposure to a person or animal (puppy or kitten) with ringworm.
RECOMMENDATION: See your dermatologist.

FINGERS AND HANDS

Your main contact with your environment is through your fingers and hands so it is not surprising that these parts of your body are open to a variety of skin diseases and conditions.

RASHES

1. **Allergy Rashes:** Redness, itching, and often small water blisters. May be due to exposure to harsh chemicals (soaps, detergents, oven cleaners, paints, polishes, greases, waxes, abrasives, turpentine, gasoline, hair-straightening products, etc.); nickel and other metals in jewelry, eyeglasses, tools and appliances, furniture, zippers, hairpins, coins, rings, etc.; sprays, perfumes, nail polish, glues, rubber, plastics, dyes, cutting oils, greases, cement, fertilizers; benzocaine, neomycin, lanolin, and other medications (even when you're just applying them on someone else); dentures; soiled diapers; and fruits and vegetables that you may handle. The list is endless, and you yourself must be the detective. [*See page 84*]

2. **Scabies:** Intense itching, mainly at night. May be accompanied by itching on wrists, fingerwebs, and genital region. [*See page 77*]

RECOMMENDATION: See your dermatologist.

3. **Eczema:** Red, weeping, itching areas and often small water blisters. May have itchy rash in bends of elbows and behind knees. [*See page 49*]

4. **Psoriasis:** Thick, silvery-white, scaly patches. May have similar patches on the elbows, knees, and scalp. [*See page 54*]

5. **Ringworm:** Well-demarcated, itchy, round or oval patch with a red border and clear center. Check for exposure to person or animal (puppy or kitten) with ringworm.

RECOMMENDATION: See your dermatologist.

6. **Vitiligo:** Depigmented patches common on the tops of the hands (almost never on the palms). May have similar depigmented areas elsewhere on the body. [*See page 141*]

TUMORS

1. **Warts:** Grayish or flesh-colored growths of varying size which may be single or in groups. [*See page 46*]

2. **Foreign Bodies:** Splinters, glass, thorns, etc. that commonly get stuck in the fingers and hands.

RECOMMENDATION: Since infection and pain may develop from these foreign bodies, it is best to see a dermatologist.

TRUNK (CHEST, ABDOMEN, BACK)
  RASHES
    1. **Acne:** Pimples and pustules, and often cysts and scars. Almost always accompanied by acne on the face. [*See page 39*]
    2. **Allergy Rashes:** Redness, itching, and occasional, small, itchy blisters. May be due to contact from clothing, soaps, detergents, fabric softener, or cosmetics (on you or on a close friend.) [*See page 84*]
    3. **Seborrheic Dermatitis:** Scaling, itching, and redness usually over the middle of the chest. May be accompanied by dandruff, and redness and scaling on the sides of the nose. [*See page 102*]
    4. **Eczema:** Red, weeping, itchy rash. Often accompanied by similar rash in the bends of the elbows and behind the knees. [*See page 49*]
    5. **Hives:** Small or large, itchy welts which appear suddenly. Similar hives may appear elsewhere on the body. May be due to a new medication, a recent penicillin injection, aspirin, a new food, or numerous other factors. [*See page 79*]
    6. **Insect Bites:** Itchy "bumps" which are very common in the summertime and often due to mosquitoes. [*See page 72*]
    7. **Pityriasis Rosea:** Pale-rose, oval patches that begins with a "herald" patch, followed by a Christmas tree-like pattern. Usually not itchy. [*See page 82*]
    8. **Shingles:** An itchy, painful rash with water blisters on one side of the body only. [*See page 67*]
    RECOMMENDATION: See your dermatologist.
    9. **Tinea Versicolor:** A "friendly" fungous infection of the skin characterized by fawn-colored, scaly patches over the chest and back. [*See page 175*]
    10. **Psoriasis:** Thick, silvery-white, scaly patches. May have similar patches over the elbows, knees, and scalp. Usually does not itch. [*See page 54*]
    11. **Vitiligo:** Depigmented, non-itchy patches that can occur on any portion of the trunk. [*See page 141*]
    12. **Ichthyosis:** Dry, fishskin-like, scaly eruption, often accompanied by a similar rash over the neck and extremities. [*See page 177*]

TUMORS
1. **Moles:** Flesh-colored, tan, or brown growths of varying size, with or without hairs. [*See page 201*]
RECOMMENDATION: See your dermatologist for any change in a mole.
2. **Dimple Warts:** Small, pearly nodules with a central depression, or bellybutton. Can occur on any portion of the trunk. Often seen in wrestlers. [*See page 168*]
RECOMMENDATION: See your dermatologist, since these small tumors are contagious.

PUBIC AREA
RASHES
1. **Seborrheic Dermatitis:** Scaling, redness, and itching. May have similar rash on the sides of the nose along with excessive dandruff. [*See page 102*]
2. **Lice ("Crabs"):** Intense itching. Check for eggs (nits) attached to the hairs as well as with intimate friends with similar itching. [*See page 75*]

TUMORS
1. **Dimple Warts:** Small, pearly nodules with a central depression, or 'bellybutton.' Very common in the pubic area. [*See page 168*]
RECOMMENDATION: See your dermatologist, since these small tumors are contagious.

PENIS AND SCROTUM
RASHES
1. **Cold Sores (herpes):** Small, itchy blisters on a red base. [*See page 61*]
2. **Allergy Rashes:** Redness, itching, and occasional, small water blisters. May be a result of exposure soaps, detergents, condoms, vaginal cream, athletic supporters, or numerous other factors. [*See page 84*]
3. **Scabies:** Intense itching, particularly at night. May have nodules on the tip of the penis and itching on wrists and between fingers. [*See page 77*]
RECOMMENDATION: See your dermatologist.
4. **Psoriasis:** Thick, reddish, scaly patches. May have similar silvery-white patches on the elbows, knees, and scalp. [*See page 54*]

5. **Lichen Planus:** Itchy, violet-colored, slightly-raised bumps on the tip of the penis. May have similar eruption on the inside of the wrists and ankles. [See page 179]

TUMORS
1. **Warts:** Flesh-colored or grayish growths. Very common on the penis. [See page 46]
2. **Dimple Warts:** Small, pearly nodules with a central depression, or 'bellybutton.' [See page 168]
RECOMMENDATION: Since these are contagious tumors, see your dermatologist.

VULVA (FEMALE GENITALS)
RASHES
1. **Allergy Rashes:** Redness, itching, and occasional, small water blisters. May be due to soaps, detergents, fabric softeners, feminine hygiene sprays, contraceptive creams, or various other irritants. [See page 84]
2. **Herpes:** Small, itchy blisters on a red base. [See page 61]
3. **Yeast Infection:** Itching and a yellowish discharge.
RECOMMENDATION: See your gynecologist.
4. **Psoriasis:** Red, scaly patches which may itch. May have similar patches on elbows, knees, and scalp. [See page 54]

TUMORS
1. **Warts:** Highly-contagious, grayish growths of varying size. Very common in the vulvar area and called condylomata acuminata. [See page 46]
RECOMMENDATION: See your dermatologist.
2. **Dimple Warts:** Small, flesh-colored, pearly nodules with a central depression, or bellybutton. [See page 168]
RECOMMENDATION: Since these are contagious tumors, see your dermatologist.

BUTTOCKS
RASHES
1. **Allergy Rashes:** Redness, itching, and occasional, small water blisters. May be due to clothing, soaps, detergents, fabric softeners, or a host of other contactants. [See page 84]
2. **Ringworm:** Well-demarcated, itchy, round or oval, scaly patches with red borders and clear centers. Check for exposure to person or animal (puppy or kitten) with ringworm.
RECOMMENDATION: See your dermatologist.

3. **Herpes:** Small, itchy water blisters on a reddened base. [*See page 61*]

4. **Psoriasis:** Thick, silvery-white, scaly patches. Usually not itchy. May have similar patches on the elbows, knees, and scalp. [*See page 54*]

RECTAL AREA
RASHES

1. **Rectal Itch:** Severe, relentless itching which is often unrelieved by any medications. Check for new toilet paper, soap, fabric softener. Any dietary changes? Any emotional problems? [*See page 185*]

2. **Psoriasis:** Red, scaly, itchy patches. May have thick, silvery-white, scaly patches on elbows, knees, and scalp. [*See page 54*]

3. **Ringworm:** Red, scaly, itchy patches often associated with athlete's foot (ringworm of the feet). [*See page 171*]

RECOMMENDATION: See your dermatologist, since ringworm infections are contagious.

TUMORS

1. **Warts:** Wet, grayish growths of varying size. [*See page 46*]
RECOMMENDATION: See your dermatologist.

THIGHS AND GROINS
RASHES

1. **Allergy Rashes:** Redness, itching, and occasional, small water blisters. May be due to clothing, soaps, detergents, fabric softeners, and a variety of other irritants. [*See page 84*]

2. **Eczema:** Red, weeping, itchy and sometimes crusted areas. May have itchy rash in the bends of the elbows and behind knees. [*See page 49*]

3. **Shingles:** Itchy, painful rash with blisters occurring on one side only. [*See page 67*]

RECOMMENDATIONS: See your dermatologist.

4. **Ringworm:** Well-demarcated, itchy, round or oval, scaly patches with red borders and clear centers. Often accompanied by athlete's foot. [*See Jock Itch, page 173*]

TUMORS

1. **Dimple Warts:** Small, flesh-colored, pearly nodules with a central depression, or bellybutton. Common in wrestlers. [*See page 168*]

RECOMMENDATION: Since these are contagious tumors, see your dermatologist.

2. **Warts:** Grayish or flesh-colored growths of varying size. May be solitary or multiple. [*See page 46*]

LEGS
   RASHES
   1. **Allergy Rashes:** Redness, itching, and occasional, small water blisters. Check for exposure to anything new. Clothing? Soap or detergent? Fabric softener? [*See page 84*]
   2. **Eczema:** Red, weeping, itchy rash, particularly behind the knees. May have itchy rash in the bends of the elbows. [*See page 49*]
   3. **Insect Bites:** Itchy bumps which hare very common in the summertime. Due to exposure to mosquitoes, fleas, or other insects. May have similar rash on other areas of body. [*See page 72*]
   4. **Ringworm:** Well-demarcated, itchy, round or oval patches with red borders and clear centers. Check for exposure to person or animal (puppy or kitten) with ringworm.
   RECOMMENDATION: See your dermatologist.
   5. **Ichthyosis:** Dry, fishskin-like, rough scales accompanied by a similar eruption over the trunk and arms. [*See page 177*]

   TUMOR
   Moles: Flesh-colored, tan, or brown growths of varying size. May or may not have hair growing in them. [*See page 201*]
   RECOMMENDATION: See your dermatologist if there has been any change in size, color, or texture.

FEET
   RASHES
   1. **Ringworm:** The most common skin affection of the feet, characterized by either scaling and itching between the toes, itchy blisters on the sole, or the so-called "moccasin" type of ringworm. Occurs mainly in teenage and adult males. [*See page 171*]
   2. **Eczema:** Red, weeping, and itchy areas. May have similar rash in the bends of the elbows and behind the knees. [*See page 49*]
   3. **Allergy Rashes:** Redness, itching, and occasional, small water blisters. May be due to contact with a variety of materials, including shoes, slippers, loafers, tennis shoes, socks, and surface medications. [*See page 84*]
   4. **Psoriasis:** Thick, silvery-white, scaly patches. Usually does not itch. May have similar patches on the elbows, knees, and scalp. [*See page 54*]

5. **Lichen Planus:** Itchy, violet-colored, slightly-raised bumps. May have similar rash with itching on wrists and small of back. [*See page 179*]

RECOMMENDATION: See your dermatologist.

TUMORS

1. **Warts:** Painful, single or multiple growths on the sole. Very common in athletic, teen-age males. [*See page 46*]

2. **Moles:** Flesh-colored, tan, or brown growths of varying size. [*See page 201*]

RECOMMENDATION: See your dermatologist if there seems to be any change in size, color, or texture.

GENERALIZED SKIN DISORDERS

Many skin conditions can affect the entire body. These include allergy rashes, eczema, hives, psoriasis, pityriasis rosea, ichthyosis, and dry skin.

For detailed information regarding these conditions, refer to them in the index.

BLACK SKIN AND
HAIR CONDITIONS

The difference between black skin and white skin is more than just color. Black people are troubled by unique skin problems. Also, their skin reacts differently to various ailments.

Some skin disorders are more common—and more apparent—in black people: keloids, "razor bumps," vitiligo, lupus erythematosus, tinea versicolor, acne due to pomades applied to the scalp, and others. Some diseases of the skin are considered unusual or rare among black people: scabies, head lice, and rosacea are some examples of these uncommon ailments.

Many skin problems in blacks are related to cosmetics designed for use on black skin and to fashion trends that are more common among blacks. For example, the use of creams and oils to reduce ashy skin color can cause hair follicle infections of the body and scalp. Also, corn-rowing, hot-combing, and hair-straightening chemicals often lead to scalp irritation and temporary hair loss.

Some allergies seem to show up more frequently in black people, as well. The most common cause of allergic reactions in black women is an ingredient (paraphenylenediamine) used in hair dyes. Allergies to nickel can cause a rash on the earlobes from earrings and on the ears and temples from the nickel in eyeglass

frames. Black men have a tendency to develop severe and continuing allergies to chromium compounds in cement and leather.
Because of the scratching and rubbing that goes along with allergy
rashes, black skin usually thickens and develops excess pigmentation, which can become a cosmetic problem.

CARE OF BLACK SKIN

While it's true that black skin is stronger and has the physio-
logical advantage of resisting sun damage, and while it doesn't
show its age as easily as white skin, it doesn't mean that you don't
have to take good care of it. To keep black skin healthy-looking,
and to prevent the excess pigmentation that can develop on
troubled and inflamed skin, follow these guidelines:

- Don't use abrasive cleansers on your face.
- Don't use harsh detergent soaps.
- Do not squeeze pimples.
- Do not use Vaseline or pomades on your scalp or face.
- Try not to scratch or irritate your skin.

Let's look at some of the skin and hair conditions that are
common to black people.

PIGMENTATION PROBLEMS

Problems with skin pigment or color—too much or too little—
can be a real concern if you're black. They show up more and are
more apparent because of the greater contrast between the normal
and problem skin, and they last longer than pigmentary problems
in others.

Even though this may sound strange, people of *all* races have
the *same number* of color-producing cells in their skin. These cells
are called melanocytes. The melanocytes in black skin produce
more color or pigment and make it faster than white skin. Further,
they are larger, more active, and are circulated differently from
those in white skin. (See chapter on Pigment.) Because of all this,
pigmentary changes in black people are usually more obvious and
longer-lasting.

Many of the color variations in black skin are normal. For
example, black skin is lighter on the palms of the hands and soles
of the feet, and darker on the gums, the roof of the mouth, and the
inner surfaces of the cheeks. Black people often have brown or

black stripes on the nails of the thumb and index finger as well as lines of pigmentation on the upper arms.

Excessive pigmentation in black skin can be the result of a simple injury, a mild irritation, or from diseases such as acne or eczema. This extra- or hyperpigmentation shows the increased activity of the color-producing cells when the skin is injured or inflamed. It can last for months or years, which can be very traumatic.

Hyperpigmentation is often seen in young black people who are being treated for acne. Blacks usually have a reaction to the drying and peeling medications used in acne therapy. The discoloration can last for years while the patient is using lotions and creams that contain the drying ingredients.

Other skin disorders that can cause color variations in black skin are eczema, psoriasis, lichen planus, tinea versicolor, and pityriasis rosea. These same conditions, paradoxically, can also cause a loss of pigment or *hypo*pigmentation. Skin injuries and liquid nitrogen treatments used to treat warts and other tumors can also cause pigmentary changes.

While there is no easy cure for these annoying pigmentary changes, you can help some of them with cortisone-like creams and ointments which your dermatologist will be able to prescribe. Other methods include some over-the-counter preparations that are discussed in the chapter on Pigment Disorders, page 138.

ASHY SKIN

Ashy skin is a result of the body getting rid of dead skin cells. This normal shedding happens in everyone of all races. This grayish, ashy-looking skin—simply dry skin—shows up more clearly on black skin because of the contrast between the dead, dry cells on the surface and the fresh, new ones that have replaced them. It is *not* a sign of disease.

You can take care of this perfectly normal, healthy skin very easily, using the same treatment as for dry skin. (*See page 58.*) Wash with a mild, gentle soap or skin cleanser (like Cetaphil Lotion), bathe in Alpha Keri Oil, apply a moisturizer (like Keri Lotion or Sofenol 5) after your bath, and try to increase the relative humidity in your home to at least 40 percent.

DERMATOSIS PAPULOSA NIGRA

Dermatosis papulosa nigra is a condition, not a disease, seen almost exclusively in blacks. It occurs in about one-third of all black people and is twice as common in women as in men.

What does it look like? Tiny, smooth, raised, mole-like spots that appear on the face and neck that are darker than the skin around them. Resembling flat warts, they begin around the age of puberty, are inherited, can vary in number from just a few to hundreds, and become more numerous as a person gets older. They never become malignant; in other words, they are not precancerous growths.

If you have a lot of these tumors and are unhappy with the way they look, a dermatologist can remove them simply and easily with a variety of methods.

KELOIDS
(See the chapter on KELOIDS that begins on page 133)

HAIR AND SCALP CONDITIONS
HAIR LOSS AND HAIR BREAKAGE

The woolly, kinky texture of black hair is uniquely different in its shape and structure from the soft, straight, flowing hair of white people.

Some hair-grooming procedures such as curling, pressing and perming stretch and stress the hair, causing it to break off or fall out.

- Traction alopecia is a term used to describe symmetrical hair loss at the margins of the hairline; in other words a receding hairline. This condition can result from tightly-braided or twisted hairstyles, tight rollers and heated curlers, and decorative corn-rowing and dreadlocks. These can cause permanent hair loss.
- Using a hot comb on chemically-treated hair can result in hair loss over the crown or top of the head.
- Using chemical relaxers and hair straighteners improperly or too frequently can cause patchy baldness by damaging the keratin of the hair, making it brittle and easy to break off.
- Using a pick can fracture the hair shaft, again leading to hair loss.

To prevent or manage hair loss and breakage, ease the stress on your hair. This may mean changing your hair style, wearing looser braids, or using pincurls instead of rollers. Also, make sure you shampoo your hair at least once a week (I know it's often difficult), and use a protein conditioner regularly.

RAZOR BUMPS

The ingrown hairs of the beard in black men are called, technically, pseudofolliculitis barbae. Almost everyone knows what you mean, though, if you call them "razor bumps." This irritation and swelling around an ingrown hair occurs mostly in young black men because the hair and hair follicles in blacks are more curved than in whites.

Razor bumps develop when the sharp, razor-cut tips of curly hair, sharpened by frequent shaving, cut into the skin in an arc and grow inward. [*See Figure A*]

Several factors make the condition worse:

- Stretching the skin out and pulling it taut when shaving. Once the skin is released, the short hairs pull back below the surface of the skin. Because of their curve and sharp tip, they re-enter the skin and pierce the wall of the hair follicle.
- Shaving against the grain.
- Shaving with a dull blade.
- Shaving with a 2-track razor. That extra track cuts the hair below the level of the skin before it has a chance to snap back.

There are no easy solutions to this common, painful inconvenience, but here are a few hints that can help:

- The simplest answer is to grow a beard and all the bumps will disappear in about a month. Why? Because by the time the hairs are about a half-inch long (in a month or so), the natural tension will cause the ends of the hairs to spring out of the skin. [*See Figure B*]

Since you may not want a beard for the rest of your life, change your shaving routine as follows:

1. Before shaving, carefully lift out any ingrown hairs with a straight pin or a beard pick.

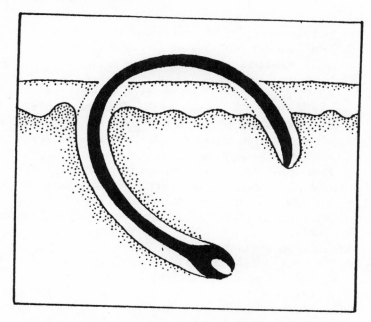

Figure A. The hair has emerged almost parallel to the skin surface, re-enters the skin, and grows downward, causing inflammation.

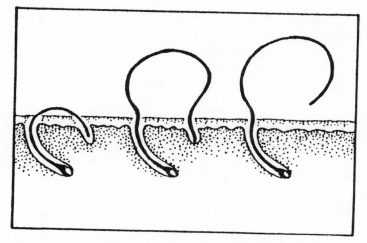

Figure B. As the hair continues to grow, the loop increases in size and pulls the tip out of the skin.

2. To soften the hairs, wash your face thoroughly with soap and hot water for at least two minutes. Rinse.
3. Apply an aerosol shaving cream and lather up for two more minutes.
4. Use only a single-edge razor.
5. Shave gently, using smooth, even strokes.
6. Shave down—one way—on the cheeks and chin.
7. Shave up—one way—on the neck.
8. Shave over one area only one time. *Do not* shave repeatedly over the same area.
9. Don't pull your beard taut when shaving.
10. Use a new razor blade every time you shave. If you can find a single-edge disposable razor, use it.
11. Shave every other day for the first two weeks, then daily.

Don't expect to get a smooth, clean shave the first few times you use this method. Be patient. After a while, you may be able to train your hairs to grow out straight, or at least straighter, rather than in a curl.

If this method doesn't work, here are a few other suggestions:

- Use a chemical depilatory. But beware—they can be irritating, they take a long time to use, they don't smell very pleasant, and they should not be used more often than every other day.
- Use electric barber clippers to shave. Since they do not cut the hair as short, they do prevent razor bumps. At the same time, though, you may not be happy with the not-as-close shave.
- Electric shavers, unfortunately, aren't much help with the problem of razor bumps.

For more information about "razor bumps," write to:
PFB Project (Pseudofolliculitis Barbae)
4801 Massachusetts Avenue, NW, Suite 400
Washington, DC 20016–2087
Robert B. Fitzpatrick, Co-Founder
202/364-8710

THE
DERMATOLOGIC
DOZEN

There are some skin disorders that are much more common than others. Acne, for example, will occur in nine out of ten youngsters, making it the most common skin ailment seen by the dermatologist—the specialist in medicine who is trained in diseases of the skin.

This chapter deals with the twelve most common dermatologic complaints—what I refer to as The Dermatologic Dozen. These occur with sufficient frequency to comprise at least 90 percent of a dermatologist's office practice.

ACNE

Acne, the scourge of adolescence, is more than skin deep. There are few skin ailments that cause as much physical and psychological anguish as this complex chemical mystery.

And there are no quick, magical cures for it.

By far the most common teenage skin disorder, acne usually begins at puberty, at a time when oil glands in the skin enlarge and increase the production of skin oil (sebum). Ranging from simple

39

pimples to angry boils, these unsightly blemishes that fall under
the general heading of acne, will plague nine out of ten pubertal
youngsters; an age when physical attractiveness becomes so important. And no one wants to be Number One on the "zit parade."

Acne appears most frequently in the mid-teens but can appears as early as the ninth year. It usually continues into the
twenties. It may appear transiently in the newborn and is often
seen in women in their mid-thirties. The condition appears earlier
in girls but is more frequent and more severe in boys. Overall,
blacks and Asians tend to have fewer and less severe acne problems.

There is a great deal of controversy concerning the causes of
acne, but most dermatologists agree that the basic problem is an
overproduction of the skin oil by enlarged oil glands. This condition is characteristic of the internal chemical changes that occur at
puberty when the skin is adjusting to a greatly increased output of
hormones.

These hormonal factors play a significant role in the onset of
acne, and since oil gland activity and sebum production are under
the control of androgens (male-type hormones), the role of these
hormones is crucial. In men the testes are the primary source of
androgenic hormones, whereas in women they are produced both
by the ovaries and the adrenal glands. Acne seems to be the result
of the oil gland's sensitivity to these androgens or their derivatives.

Acne also can be hereditary. Parents who had severe acne
during their teenage years often have children who develop severe
acne.

Acne occurs on areas of the body where oil glands are the
largest, most numerous, and most active: the face, chest, and back.
Simply stated, these enlarged and overactive oil glands become
clogged with oil and sticky skin cells, thus forming blackheads and
whiteheads. (When a skin pore is closed and oil can't escape, the
swelling is called a whitehead; when the skin pore isn't closed but
is simply plugged up with dead cells and oil, it's called a blackhead. The dark color of the blackhead is *not* due to dirt: it is a
result of pigment cells— melanin—in the upper layers of the skin.)
The glands continue to manufacture oil which is unable to escape.

Bacteria, which are always on the skin in "friendly" and
harmless numbers, set up housekeeping and begin to thrive in
these trapped secretions. They then become "unfriendly" and
harmful, causing infected pimples, or zits. These zits may lead to

cysts (little sacs filled with fluid or cheesy material), which then break down to form scars.

Many external factors can aggravate acne. Anything that prevents the oily secretions from flowing freely out of the oversized oil gland, such as infrequent washing, long hair (particularly bangs), hairspray, mousses and greasy hair dressing, and moisturizers. Other cosmetics containing lanolin can further plug up the already clogged oil gland opening to produce new lesions. Youngsters working at gas stations or fast food restaurants, who are constantly exposed to greases and oils, are especially prone to acne flare-ups.

Another type of acne—acne mechanica—is an aftermath of physical irritation to specific areas of the body, either resulting in or aggravating prior acne. A common example of this process is the development of acne over the forehead, chin and back in teenage football players as a result of wearing football helmets, chin straps, and shoulder pads. These sources of friction, combined with heavy perspiration, may cause acne lesions over the affected pressure areas.

Other factors that can aggravate acne include hormonal disorders and taking drugs such as cortisone, iodides, lithium, vitamin B12, and anti-epilepsy medications. Young men who are taking anabolic steroids for body-building are prone to the severe cystic type of acne that doesn't respond to conventional anti-acne medications. Young women often experience acne eruptions just before their menstrual periods. The "low-dose" birth control pills also are responsible for acne in women who never had the problem as adolescents. Many women note a worsening—even an onset—of acne after stopping their oral contraceptive. This phenomenon can last as long as two years.

There also is some indication that acne around the mouth is aggravated by fluoridated toothpastes. Persistent localized acne over the temples and forehead may be caused by excessive brushing with a hair brush or hair dryer attachment.

Acne usually lasts for several years and abates in the early twenties. The conflicts and tensions that may arise along the way can lead to feelings of inferiority, insecurity, and inadequacy, which undermine self-confidence. After acne has burned itself out, it may leave permanent scars on the psyche as well as on the skin. Both subside with time, but if the skin scars are severe, they may benefit from further treatment in the form of dermabrasion, chemical peel, punch grafting, or collagen injections.

While there is no easy cure for acne, you can control it to lessen its severity and to prevent the pitting and scarring that arise from neglect and self-medication.

The key to acne therapy is to control the overactivity of the oil glands, shrink them if possible, and destroy the bacteria that are responsible for the infection. And the earlier you treat your acne, the better.

Here are a few general principles that can help prevent or control acne:

- Wash your face thoroughly at least three times daily.
- Don't pick or squeeze. This may aggravate the condition and lead to infection and scarring.
- Shampoo your hair frequently.
- Keep your hair off your face and don't use hairsprays, mousses, or greasy hair dressings.
- Avoid greasy cosmetics.
- Avoid creamy suntan lotions.
- Facials are not recommended because the creams and lotions force more oil into the already clogged pores.
- If you have acne near your mouth, stop your fluoridated toothpaste for a few months and note whether it makes any difference.
- Avoid emotional stress. The chemicals released by your body during anxious and stressful situations stimulate the adrenal gland to produce more of the male-type hormone (more so in women!) which, in turn, stimulates the overproduction of skin oil.
- Watch your diet. The role that diet plays in causing acne is controversial and debatable. I recommend that you cut out chocolate, seafood, nuts, and cheeses, and that you limit milk to three glasses a day.
- If your physician has prescribed tetracycline for your acne, do not take multiple-vitamin supplements containing iron. Iron interferes with the absorption of tetracycline.

No therapy really "cures" acne. New lesions can occur despite good management. It can be controlled, however, to lessen its severity and to prevent the scarring that may result. Don't be discouraged if your progress is slow. If you are diligent, conscientious, and faithful with your treatment, you will reap the benefit of a clearer complexion.

It is especially important that parents try to understand their teenagers' plight. By offering encouragement and helping your teenager maintain his or her self-esteem, you can help lessen the mental anguish and psychological scars that so often accompany acne.

Every day brings promise of a new magical cure. The latest heralded treatment for acne is an oral drug of the vitamin A family, 13-*cis*-retinoic acid. Sold under the name Accutane, this rather expensive prescription medication works by shrinking the oil glands to reduce the output of skin oil.

The Food and Drug Administration has approved Accutane for only the very severe and stubborn form of cystic acne which generally doesn't respond well to conventional forms of medication. Many dermatologists fear that it will be prescribed improperly and injudiciously by well-meaning but overeager general physicians for the common, garden-variety type of acne.

Accutane has many drawbacks. Pregnant women should not take Accutane because of the possibility of defects in the newborn. And women of childbearing age must show proof that they are not pregnant when they begin a course of Accutane treatments.

Accutane may also cause various undesirable side effects, including chapped lips, dry nose, dry mouth, dry skin, nosebleeds, and generalized itching. Other adverse reactions include muscular aches and pains, fatigue, headaches, conjunctivitis, blurred vision, and hair loss. These side effects are all temporary, and disappear when the drug is discontinued.

Also, during Accutane therapy, blood tests must be taken every two or three weeks to determine the level of certain fatty substances—triglycerides—which often become elevated during therapy.

If your acne is stubborn, persistent, and disfiguring, consult your dermatologist. Waiting to "outgrow" acne can be a serious mistake; permanent scarring can result if acne is left untreated. A dermatologist can prescribe internal and topical medications to eliminate or lighten this cross that almost all teenagers have to bear.

COMMON MYTHS AND MISCONCEPTIONS
Myth #1: Acne is a disease of adolescence.

While it is true that acne usually appears during puberty, this is not always the case. Many people, particularly women, don't develop acne until their twenties or thirties, and it can afflict both men and women well into their forties.

Myth #2: Acne is more common in girls.

Young women are more likely to see a dermatologist about their acne problems because, as a rule, they are more conscious of their appearance. However, acne affects both sexes equally. As a matter of fact, the severe cystic form of acne of the back is more common in men.

Myth #3: Acne is due to improper hygiene.

In reality, acne patients generally are more fastidious and conscientious about cleanliness than other teenagers. Blackheads, the primary hallmark of acne, do not result from dirt but from pigment (melanin) in the oil glands.

Myth #4: Masturbation causes or aggravates acne.

The only link between masturbation and acne is that both are often associated with adolescence. Moralists of the 19th century blamed many diseases on such "sinful" practices. The guilt surrounding masturbation in the minds of many teenagers probably perpetuates this timeworn myth.

Myth #5: Sexual intercourse will cure acne.

While this form of therapy sounds appealing, there is no evidence to document that it works. This belief probably stems from an old European myth that marriage cures acne. People often got married in their early twenties, about the same time that acne usually burns itself out.

TREATING ACNE

The following is a list of some of the specific measures and products I recommend to reduce, eliminate, or "mask" zits and other acne lesions. There are countless products available for controlling acne, and new products are being developed all the time. I have limited this list to a few of those products that many dermatologists recommend and that give my patients best results.

Wash your face thoroughly at least three times a day. For mild acne, where there are mainly blackheads and some oiliness, use either:

Fostex Medicated Cleansing Bar (Westwood)

Sal-Ac Acne Cleanser (GenDerm)

For the more severe types of acne, when you need extra degreasing, try either:

Fostex 10% Benzoyl Peroxide Wash (Westwood)

PanOxyl Bar 5% or 10% (Stiefel)

Clearasil DoubleClear Pads (Richardson-Vicks)

For mild acne apply either of the following to the pimples once or twice daily:

Fostril Lotion (Westwood)

Rezamid Lotion (Dermik)

For more severe acne, try any of the following benzoyl peroxide preparations:

Clear by Design (SmithKline)

BenOxyl Lotion 5% (Stiefel)

Vanoxide Lotion (Dermik)

Fostex 10% Benzoyl Peroxide Gel (Westwood)

These preparations should cause slight peeling to help dry up your pimples. If your face gets too dry, use the products less often. If your face beings to itch, burn, or turn red, you may be allergic to one of the ingredients. Stop the medication, and apply cool, wet compresses to your face. Do not use the medication again; use a different or milder preparation.

If your face is very greasy, use one of the following astringents several times a day to remove the excess oil that accumulates:

Drytex (C&M Pharmacal)

Seba-Nil Liquid Cleanser (Owen)

The following are a few "therapeutic" makeups and cover-ups you can use to mask and heal your acne lesions:

Acnotex Lotion (C&M Pharmacal)

Fostex Medicated Cover-up (Westwood)

Liquimat Lotion (Owen) - available in several different shades.

Shampoo daily, if possible. Patients with acne usually have oily hair. When too much oil collects on the scalp and hair, it gets onto your face and further plugs up the already clogged oil glands. An interesting phenomenon is that young women (and men) with unusually long hair—no matter how they style it—very often have acne on their backs.

For exceptionally oily hair use any of the following:

Pernox Shampoo (Westwood)

Ionil Shampoo (Owen)

DHS Shampoo (Person & Covey)

Keep your hair off your face, eliminate bangs, and avoid hair-sprays, mousses, and greasy hair dressings. Use creme rinses in moderation.

Avoid greasy cosmetics. An oil-free, water-based cosmetic cover-up is the best type of make-up even for those who do *not* have acne problems.

Here are a couple of the better cover-ups, that are less likely to cause or aggravate acne:

Pore Minimizer or *Stay-True Makeup* (Clinique)

Demi-Matte Makeup (Estee Lauder)

In addition, Owen/Allercreme and Almay manufacture a complete line of oil-free makeups for acne patients. Try one. Try all. Only you can decide what's best for you.

If you need a moisturizer, the only acceptable ones I recommend are:

Candermyl (Owen/Galderma)

Moisturel (Westwood)

Colladerm Gel (C&M Pharmacal)

Note: If you have acne on one cheek only, or more on one cheek, you may have the habit of resting that cheek on your palm while talking on the telephone, or while asleep. Try to break the habit.

WARTS

Over 20 million people in this country have warts. The common myth that they are caused by handling frogs or toads is, of course, only a myth. Frogs and toads have their own problems. Warts are growths on the skin caused by viruses. They should be destroyed because they are contagious, unsightly, and occasionally painful.

You can pass warts on to others by direct or indirect contact, in such places as locker rooms, public shower stalls, gymnasium mats, and swimming pools. Very often, members of the same household are afflicted with warts. They can also spread on the same person by picking, scratching, shaving, or biting one's nails.

Warts come in many shapes and sizes and can turn up on different parts of the body. The so-called common wart is a raised, rough, grayish-looking, painless growth. It can vary in size from a pinhead to a fairly large mass. While they may occur on any portion of the skin surface and mucous membranes, common warts are usually found on the fingers, hands, and soles of the feet.

Flat warts are smooth, flesh-colored, and slightly-elevated. These matchhead-size growths usually appear on the face and backs of hands of children and young adults. Genital warts are found in the moist areas of the genital and anal regions.

Warts on the sole are called plantar warts. (Not "planter's warts," as some people are fond of saying, as if there were something agricultural or occupational about them.) These warts are the most stubborn variety and frequently resist all known treatments.

That there are dozens of widely proclaimed methods to eliminate warts attests to the fact that there is no single predictably effective remedy. Ideally, the treatment should be quick, safe, and painless. And it should produce no unsightly or lasting scars.

Some doctors recommend that the best way to manage warts is to let them manage themselves. If left untreated, many warts will disappear by themselves in about two years. This seems to be the natural history of warts. Warty people, however, may not want to wait for any spontaneous cure, and so they seek medical advice.

Methods that physicians use to treat warts are about as varied as warts themselves. The type of treatment your doctor uses will depend upon your age, the location of your warts, and the size and number of warts to be treated.

In electrosurgery the wart is burned off with an electric needle under a local anesthetic. Warts also can be chemically destroyed using various types of acids, plasters, and other chemicals. Other warts can be frozen off using liquid nitrogen at minus 320 degrees Fahrenheit. Still other warts succumb to surgical excision (cutting the wart out under local anesthesia). A less widely used method is X-ray therapy carefully administered by a dermatologist. In selected cases, such as stubborn plantar warts, this method can produce miracles. Recent concern over the effects of radiation, however, has restricted its use. One of the latest modes of therapy for large or stubborn warts is the argon laser.

Genital and anal warts are usually transmitted by sexual contact and it is essential to treat the patient's sexual partner to prevent recurrences. These venereal-type warts respond to podophyllin—a resinous substances that a physician paints on the warty growths at weekly intervals.

Some doctors (and some grandmothers) charm warts away by suggestive methods. These "witching" methods have worked in many individuals, particularly young, impressionable children, and they leave no scars, no matter how deep or long-standing the warts may have been. Regardless of how bizarre or ludicrous a treatment may sound, if the patient has faith in the "charmer," the warts usually will disappear. (However, I do not recommend stealing a piece of beef or a dishrag!)

A great deal of research is going on to determine why certain people get warts, why others do not, and why warts often disap-

Exorcism

For stubborn warts around and under the finger-nails, use the following method, which I call "ad-hesotherapy":

Completely wrap the wart with four layers of plain adhesive tape. (See Figure) Don't wrap too tightly!

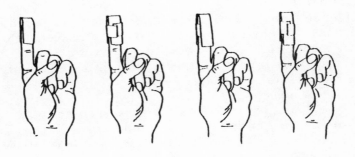

Figure. Wrap the wart completely with four layers of adhesive tape as shown above and make it airtight. Leave on for 6½ days. Remove for half a day. Repeat the entire procedure (6½ days on, ½ day off). After 3 or 4 weeks, the wart "gets tired" and disappears, leaving no scar.

pear spontaneously. In the meantime, if you can't ward off warts, take comfort in knowing that your doctor can help you get rid of them.

TREATING WARTS

For small, flat warts of the face and the backs of the hands, ask your pharmacist for the following:

Castor Oil (one ounce)

Directions: Apply to warts twice daily using a cotton-tipped applicator (Q-Tip).

For the common type of warts on your fingers, palms, feet, and other areas, use either:

Dr. Scholl's Wart Medicine

Compound W Gel (Whitehall)

Directions: Apply to warts at night. Do not cover. Discontinue if irritation occurs.

FOLKLORE REMEDIES FOR WARTS

Take a dead black cat to a graveyard at midnight. When you hear a noise, throw the cat toward the sound. That will take the warts away.

Steal a greasy dishrag from your neighbor. Wipe your warts with it, then throw it over your left shoulder into a pond.

Rub warts with a raw potato, then bury the potato in clay. Just to be on the safe side, repeat with another potato the following day.

Rub warts with a black snail and impale the snail on a thorn tree. When the snail dries and withers, so do the warts.

Rub the warts with a chicken gizzard during the waning of the moon. Then bury the gizzard in the center of a dirt road.

Rub warts with a cinder, wrap the cinder up in paper, and leave it at a crossroads. Whoever picks up the parcel and unwraps it, catches the warts.

Prick the wart with a gooseberry thorn passed through a wedding ring.

Lick your forefinger and point it at a passing funeral three times and say, "My warts go with you."

Rub the wart with a piece of stolen beef. Then bury the meat.

ECZEMA

Itch . . . scratch. . . .

Itch . . . scratch . . . scratch. . . .

In brief, this is the story of what people frequently call "eczema" and what dermatologists call "atopic dermatitis." It is the disease that starts from scratch and one that may last a lifetime. It is the eczema of infancy, the chronic, relentless dermatitis of childhood and adolescence, and the fierce and uncontrollable itching of the adult.

Eczema is a general term which, to most people, means a diffuse rash with itching. It is a synonym for dermatitis, which literally means "inflammation of the skin."

But when physicians speak of eczema, they usually refer to the persistent, incessant itchy eruption that almost invariably begins in infancy, is inherited, is often accompanied in later years by hay fever or asthma, and in rare circumstances lasts a lifetime. It is atopic dermatitis, a disease that affects about 10 millions people in the United States alone.

No one yet knows the "why" of this virtually uncontrollable, allergic process. It begins with itching on a perfectly normal looking skin. You then rub, claw, tear, and scratch where it itches and you, yourself, produce the rash we know of as eczema.

There are three different types or "stages" of atopic dermatitis.

The infantile form. This usually begins about six or eight weeks after birth. The itching is often intense and lasts up until about the age of two years. The rash, which almost always affects the cheeks and mouth, usually worsens after vaccinations and immunization injections and during the teething phase. During the second year of life, the itchy areas develop over the hands, wrists, and outer portions of the arms and legs.

The childhood type. While the infantile form in over half the cases fades out between the ages of two and four, it may continue into the so-called childhood type of eczema. The areas that suffer most here are the creases in the elbows and the bends of the knees. The affected areas are more dry, the skin becomes thicker and grayish in color, the itching becomes fierce, and the children are restless, anxious, and hyperactive.

Of all the eczemas that occur during childhood, atopic dermatitis is not only the most prevalent disorder, but it is also one of the most mystifying and difficult to manage.

The adolescent and adult types. The infantile and childhood eczemas often disappear after a few years only to reappear in late adolescence. While it usually fades away by the age of thirty, it may persist throughout the entire lifetime of some unfortunate person. The itching, again, may be intense and is usually worse at night. The areas affected are the bends of the elbows and knees, the face, the shoulders, and the upper back. The itchy and scratched skin becomes thick and leathery, darker than the surrounding skin, and develops dry scales.

Another characteristic feature is the accentuated groove beneath the lower eyelids. This is called the atopic pleat.

The management of eczema is an enormous challenge for the physician. No one treatment for eczema works for everyone, since the areas involved and the degree of itching affect different people in different ways. At best we try to alleviate the intense itching which, in essence, *is* the disease. Interrupt and stop this fierce symptom and we break the itch-scratch reflex which is wholly responsible for the clinical manifestation—the rash.

Although there is no specific treatment for controlling eczema, here are some general rules and measures to follow:

- **Never use soap!** Soap removes the natural oils from your already overdry skin. Use a soapless cleanser, such as *Cetaphil Lotion*, or a soap substitute, such as *Lowila Cake.*
- Take baths and showers in lukewarm—not hot—water. Add soothing bath oils to the water for excessively dry, scaly skin. And when you dry, dry by patting—not by rubbing.
- Keep fingernails short and clean.
- Avoid sudden extremes of temperature and any violent exercise that causes sweating. Going from a hot to a cold or from a cold to a hot environment will trigger the itching mechanism.
- Keep the relative humidity above 40 percent—winter and summer—to protect the already dry skin from becoming completely dehydrated.
- Eliminate fuzzy, rough, and woolen clothing as these aggravate eczema. Soft, loose, cotton clothing is best.
- Get rid of furry and fuzzy toys and feather pillows.
- Do not allow children to play on floor rugs or rough upholstery.
- And while it may seem cruel to you, removing household pets, particularly longhaired dogs and cats, is a must.
- Don't work around or expose yourself to dust, industrial chemicals, fumes, sprays, cutting oils, paints, varnishes, and solvents. All these will tend to worsen your eczema.
- Avoid all cosmetics, cleansers, body oils, and lotions that contain lanolin. Lanolin is good for sheep but bad for humans. It causes allergies, plugs up oil glands (causing acne), and aggravates eczema. (Besides, why use a product on your skin that is advertised as great for polishing shoes and cleaning pots?)
- Avoid colds and other respiratory infections. These lower the resistance of your skin and make your atopic dermatitis worse.
- Don't wear rubber gloves for household chores. Even the cotton-lined varieties "sweat" when immersed in hot water, thereby leaching out the chemicals and stabilizers in the rubber which only exacerbate eczema skin of the fingers and hands. If you find that you must do the housework and

dishes with rubber gloves, get cotton liners (*Dermal Gloves*) and wear them at all times under the cotton-lined rubber gloves.

- Avoid exposing yourself to people who have cold sores (fever blisters). The virus that causes cold sores can cause serious eruptions in people who have eczema.
- Avoid over-the-counter salves and lotions containing benzocaine and antihistamines.
- Don't use Vaseline and other greasy ointments. These tend to intensify the itching by preventing the evaporation of sweat.
- During the winter holidays, steer clear of live Christmas trees. The artificial varieties are less irritating and less allergenic to eczema sufferers.
- Whenever possible, avoid emotional stress and tension. You may find that a flare-up of your condition was actually triggered by some conflict, anxiety, or stressful situation. There is no other skin condition where "nerves" play a greater role.
- Diet is not a factor in most cases of eczema, but if you think that your rash worsens after eating a certain food, eliminate it for a few weeks to see if your condition improves. Frequently implicated foods are: milk, cheese, spices, citrus fruits, seafood, fish, and eggs.
- Try not to scratch. Not only will scratching aggravate your condition, but it can break and damage your skin, thus contributing to secondary bacterial infection.

Above all, try to be patient and keep a positive attitude. Despite the agony it can cause, eczema is not a serious disorder. If you can learn to live with it and keep the rash under control, chances are it will burn itself out of its own record.

If, however, your rash persists and the itching is uncontrollable, see your dermatologist. He or she will be able to prescribe some time-tested remedies in the form of creams, lotions, cortisone-like drugs, and, perhaps, antibiotics if your rash becomes infected.

TREATING ECZEMA

For the acute, weeping, and oozing type of eczema, soothing wet dressings and baths will relieve the inflammation and itching.

For acute, localized eczema, use the following as an open wet dressing:

Bluboro Powder (Herbert)

Directions are on the package. Use as open wet dressings as described on page 217.

For acute, widespread eczema, the best form of therapy is a soothing bath taken in any of the following bath oils:

Alpha Keri Bath Oil (Westwood)

Jeri-Bath (Dermik)

Nutraderm Bath Oil (Owen)

Directions are on the bottles.

When the weeping and oozing have begun to dry up, discontinue the wet dressings. Now you can use a cream or lotion to help relieve the itching and help the skin maintain its smoothness and resiliency. Try any of the following:

Hytone Cream 0.5% (Dermik)

Sarna Lotion (Stiefel)

Schamberg's Lotion (C&M Pharmacal)

Directions: Apply every 3 or 4 hours and after your bath.

For the dry, scaly, chronic variety of eczema, where the skin is tight and thickened, you may try the following lubricating preparation:

Cort-Aid Ointment (Upjohn)

For generalized, chronic eczema use the following bath additive:

Balnetar (Westwood)

Directions for use on the bottle.

For any stage of eczema, never use soap. Use the following cleanser or soap substitute bar for all cleansing purposes:

Cetaphil Lotion (Owen)

Lowila Cake (Westwood)

For the itching that accompanies all eczema, take either of the following antihistamines every 4 hours as necessary.

Chlor-Trimeton Tablets [4 mg] (Schering)

Dimetane Tablets [4 mg] (Robins)

See directions and cautions on the labels for proper dosage.

Note: Never use any surface medications containing:

- "-caine" derivatives, the most common being benzocaine.
- Antihistamine creams and lotions such as *Benadryl, Caladryl, PBZ,* or *Ziradryl.*

For more information about eczema, write to:
National Eczema Society
Travistock House North
London WC1H 9SR
UK 01–388–4097
C.M. Funnel, Coordinator

PSORIASIS

"But Naaman's leprosy [psoriasis] will cling to you and your descendants forever." And Gehazi left his presence a leper, white as now.

2 Kings 5:27

Psoriasis is a stubborn, chronic, and as yet incurable disease of the skin. Some eight million people suffer from psoriasis in the United States alone. And they spend more than $1 billion a year ($2,000 every minute!) to treat this poorly understood ailment.

Psoriasis—the word comes from the Greek *psora* which means itch—was considered a form of leprosy in biblical times. But this "disease of healthy people" doesn't threaten or shorten lives. It is neither an infection nor an allergy. It probably is not due to any vitamin or mineral deficiency. It doesn't leave scars or make you lose your hair. And, except in severe cases, it doesn't interfere with physical activities. (In fact, it may not even itch). To the psoriasis sufferer, however, it can be an emotionally disabling and traumatic disorder.

Psoriasis is characterized by patches of raised, red skin covered by silvery-white scales. It can occur at any age, but commonly begins in young adulthood. It usually recurs at unpredictable intervals and may be worse in the winter. It is often precipitated or aggravated by physical or emotional stress, upper respiratory infections, strep throat, alcoholic beverages, obesity, certain oral medications (lithium and anti-malarial drugs are but a few), and skin injuries such as scratches, cuts, and burns, including sunburn.

Psoriasis is not contagious. It does seem to run in families—about one-third of psoriatic patients have a family history of the condition—although the pattern of heredity is not clear. It is also associated with a form of arthritis which affects the joints of the fingers.

No one knows the cause of psoriasis, but we do know how it comes about. Normal skin cells have a life span of about twenty-eight days. This is the time it takes for a cell to be born, move to the outer surface of the skin, and flake off.

In psoriasis, due to some abnormality in the mechanism which makes the skin grow and replace itself, this orderly process goes awry. The skin cells turn over at a rate ten times faster than the normal cells, causing a build-up of scales in thick, red, and sharply-bordered patches. These patches may be small, the size of a matchhead or smaller, or extremely large, covering the entire body. If these patches appear in the body's creases and folds, they may cause itching and pain. Although psoriasis can affect any part of the skin, the patches usually occur on the elbows, knees, and scalp.

Psoriasis comes in many shapes and forms. It can, for example, limit itself to the fingernails and toenails as small pits or stippling or loosening of the nails from their beds. In some unfortunate people, it affects the genital area and can limit sexual activity. In extreme cases it is widespread, with total body redness and scaling, causing severe embarrassment which, in turn, can lead to psychological problems: the true "heartbreak" of psoriasis.

If you have psoriasis, there are some remedies you can try yourself. But for serious or stubborn cases, I recommend you see your dermatologist. There are many treatments, both old and new, that require a doctor's know-how.

The method of treatment depends on the extent and severity of the symptoms. An old standby is one of the various types of tar preparations which have been used with good results by thousands of psoriasis sufferers. Other methods are sunlight and ultraviolet radiation. There are also cortisone-like medications that are applied or injected into the patches as well as various oral remedies which, while often effective, may have potentially serious side effects. One of these is methotrexate, a drug that has been used for many years to treat difficult and extensive cases of psoriasis. Treatment with methotrexate is complicated by nausea, mouth ulcers, headaches, and harmful effects on the liver.

The latest powerful oral medication for severe and stubborn psoriasis is a pill called etretinate (*Tegison*). It is extremely effective for the severe, generalized forms of psoriasis, but there are many serious, adverse side effects. If you plan to enter into this therapy, make sure your dermatologist explains it to you.

Every new treatment for psoriasis becomes headline news.

Most of these "miracle treatments" quickly fall into disfavor or are discarded when another "breakthrough" is heralded. One of the popular treatments, PUVA therapy, is aimed at slowing down excess cell reproduction. The patient swallows a harmless drug called methoxsalen and then is exposed to longwave ultraviolet light. The proponents of this therapy swear by it, and today it has become a fashionable treatment for people with extensive psoriasis. There is some indication, however, that the PUVA treatment can lead to severe skin damage appearing many years later. Another reported treatment, called climatotherapy, consists of bathing in the Dead Sea!

But let's face it. While many of these treatments can help relieve the itching and scaling, there is no known "cure" for psoriasis. The cure will come about only when we know the exact nature and mechanism of the disease.

And while you must face the possibility that psoriasis will be a permanent guest in your life, let me offer some general guidelines to help you overcome the difficulties that accompany your condition:

- Avoid emotional stress and tension.
- Try not to worry about what you consider the unsightly appearance of your rash. (It looks a lot worse to you than it does to other people.)
- If it itches, try not to scratch.
- Avoid those widely advertised "quick cures."
- While diet plays only a small role in psoriasis, I recommend that you limit your intake of red meat, poultry, eggs, dairy products, and alcoholic beverages for a few weeks to see if it helps. I know that doesn't leave much, but a temporary diet of fish and vegetables is a small price to pay for the chance of relief.
- Cooperate with your dermatologist.
- Don't be discouraged if progress is slow.
- And take comfort in knowing that with the variety of medications and treatments available, this potentially traumatic and hopeless disorder has a good chance of being controlled.

TREATING PSORIASIS

Since psoriasis remains a chronic disease with no cure currently available, management focuses on controlling the visible features, the flakes and scales, of the disorder. And while there is no reliable, sure-fire treatment for psoriasis, you often can relieve the scaling and itching that accompany it.

For generalized or widespread psoriatic patches, tar baths are very helpful, provided you are not allergic to tar. Try any of the following tar preparations in your bath:

Balnetar (Westwood)

Lavatar (Doak)

Polytar Bath (Stiefel)

Directions for use are on the bottles.

Various tar medications can be very helpful in controlling localized patches of psoriasis. They are safer and less expensive than the strong cortisone-type preparations. However, they all stink, sting, and stain. The following are two of the more popular and effective tar preparations.:

Estar Gel (Westwood)

PsoriGel (Owen)

Directions for each are on the labels.

Note: Never apply tar preparations to inflamed skin and avoid contact with the eyes. In rare instances, either of the above may cause some type of allergy.

For psoriasis of the scalp, a stubborn area to treat, it is important to shampoo often (daily or twice daily!) and thoroughly. Effective shampoos include those with tar. Try any of the following and find out which is best for you:

Ionil-T Shampoo (Owen)

Duplex-T Shampoo (C&M Pharmacal)

DHS Tar Gel Shampoo (Person & Covey)

Polytar Shampoo (Stiefel)

To lessen scalp involvement, avoid even minimal injuries that can arise from metal combs, stiff brushes, tight curlers, picking, and scratching.

If your scalp condition is stubborn, use any of the following lotions:

SLT Lotion (C&M Pharmacal)

T/Gel Scalp Solution (Neutrogena)

P&S Liquid (Baker/ Cummins)

Directions for each are on the labels.

About 85% of people with psoriasis benefit from sunlight. Fifteen percent either get worse or are not affected at all by exposure to the sun.

Some people improve by restricting certain foods and beverages, especially seafood, liquor, and beer. Some drugs, taken internally, such as lithium, also aggravate psoriasis. If you think something is making your psoriasis worse, be a detective and eliminate the culprit.

For more information concerning psoriasis, write to:

National Psoriasis Foundation
6442 SW Beaverton Highway, Suite 201
Portland, Oregon 97221
503/297–1545
Gail M. Zimmerman, Executive Director

DRY SKIN

June 8, 1955

Found Winston in his bath in his most unreasonable mood.

"This tickle," he grunted, "is quite intolerable. It kept me awake. Yes, a bloody night. The skin man has given me fourteen ointments or lotions in turn without any theory behind any of them. Just doling out some potion or unguent to keep me quiet. It's a disgrace to the medical faculty."

As the tenure of office of Winston's adviser seemed to be threatened, I had to explain to Winston that his skin had grown old with the rest of his tissues, and that none of us could put back the clock. He gave an impatient snort. He was not convinced. I explained to him that if he were willing to cut down the number of hot baths it might help the irritation of his skin very considerably. This he regarded as an outrageous suggestion.

Winston Churchill. Taken from *Diaries of Lord Moran.* (Boston: Houghton Mifflin, 1966.)

Thus wrote Lord Moran about Sir Winston Churchill's intolerable and protracted dry skin itch.

Dry skin is a loose, unscientific term used to describe rough, scaly, and flaky skin—most often on areas below the neck—that is dry to the touch and less flexible or elastic than normal skin. And lest you think otherwise, let me set the record straight: dry skin does *not* cause wrinkles.

Dryness of the skin usually develops as winter approaches. When the temperature drops and the relative humidity decreases, the upper layers of your skin lose a large amount of water. This leads to dry skin with its scaling and occasional itching.

This lowered humidity is further aggravated by artificial heating which, in addition to warming the air, dries it. The dry, heated air expands like a sponge, sucking up moisture from objects in the area, such as plants (which begin to wither), furniture (which begins to crack), and our skin. We usually notice the drop in relative humidity when we get those unexpected shocks from a build-up of static electricity.

Dry skin has a tendency to improve automatically during the summer months because perspiration keeps the skin moist as it reaches the skin surface. When there is high relative humidity, there's less evaporation of moisture from our skin.

Dermatologists used to think that dry skin was caused entirely by a lack of oily film on the surface of the skin. We now know that it's due to water loss from the skin's outer layers and to the inability of moisture to move from the deeper layers to the surface. While the natural oils on the skin surface protect the water from evaporating from the lower layers, these oils really can't prevent dry skin if there isn't enough moisture in the cells to begin with.

Several factors influence dry skin. It is more common in the elderly where, despite adequate water content of the skin, there are diminished oily secretions. Using harsh, alkaline soaps and soaking too long and too often in very hot baths can do it. Overheated homes with low humidity, as well as air-conditioning (which also lowers the relative humidity), likewise contribute to dry skin. Other factors include too much sunbathing, overexposure to wind and cold, fuzzy and woolen clothing, towels and sheets that you may have laundered in harsh detergents but not rinsed well enough, and nutritional problems resulting from poor diet.

Here are some general guidelines for avoiding dry skin:

- Increase the relative humidity in your home to at least 40 percent by properly adjusting the heating or air-conditioning systems. If this is not practicable, buy a good, commercial room humidifier.
- When you bathe or shower, don't use extremely hot water or harsh soaps.
- Avoid excessive sunbathing, cold temperatures, and strong winds.

- Don't wear heavy, woolen, fuzzy clothing.
- Keep healthy, make sure you eat a well-balanced diet, and drink plenty of water.

If you suffer from dry skin, try switching to mild gentle soaps and use soothing bath oils and water-attracting creams and lotions that keep in your skin's natural moisture and leave it smooth, soft, and supple.

TREATING DRY SKIN

Judging from the number of ads on TV and in magazines for products promising relief of dry skin, everyone in this country must suffer at some time from this condition. The products used to treat dry skin of the body include bath oils, emollient creams and lotions, and soaps.

Since skin dryness results from lack of water, an excellent way to replace this loss is by bathing in water that has a bath oil in it. These coat the body and seal in the needed moisture to plump up the skin cells and make the skin more soft and pliable. (CAUTION: All bath oils make the tub surface slippery. Be very careful getting in and out of the tub. They also make the tub hard to clean, so you'll have to give it a good scrubbing with cleanser when you're finished.)

I suggest you try any of the following bath oils:

Alpha Keri Bath Oil (Westwood)

Jeri-Bath (Dermik)

Nutraderm Bath Oil (Owen)

Directions for use are on each bottle.

The following emollient preparations help soften and lubricate the skin:

Moisturel Lotion (Westwood)

Sofenol-5 (C&M Pharmacal)

Shepard's Cream Lotion (Dermik)

LactiCare Lotion (Stiefel)

Directions for use on each container.

The following moisturizing preparations contain special ingredients to treat excessive dryness of the body, relieve itching, and help make the skin more supple and springy:

NutraPlus Lotion (Owen)

Aquacare/HP Lotion (Herbert)

Directions for use on each container.

Avoid harsh soaps which tend to strip the oils from the skin surface, and try any of the following:

Alpha Keri Soap (Westwood)

Basis Soap (Beiersdorf)

Cetaphil Lotion (Owen/Galderma)

For especially dry skin of the body, when the other products don't seem to be working, try either of the following creams:

Complex 15 Cream or *Lotion* (Baker/Cummins)

Carmol-20 Cream (Syntex)

Directions for use are on the labels.

Note: I do not recommend any of the aforementioned creams and lotions for use on the face. They will only plug up oil glands and cause whiteheads and blackheads.

COLD SORES AND GENITAL HERPES

"O'er ladies' lips, who straight on kisses dream,
  Which oft the angry Mab with blisters plagues,
  Because their breaths with sweetmeats tainted are."

Shakespeare, *Romeo and Juliet*, 1.4.74

Like the common cold, cold sores are frequent, worldwide, and unresponsive to present-day treatments. They are also highly contagious, the infection being spread primarily through social and sexual activities, usually involving close person-to-person contact. This, particularly in the case of genital herpes, can be most distressing.

Some people became infected from contact with eating and drinking utensils, from towels, and—yes—even from toilet seats! Close body contact in wrestling, rugby, and other sports can transmit the disease, and health care personnel are at special risk for infection of their fingers. Fortunately, cold sores are more irritating than they are dangerous.

The typical cold sore consists of a small group of water blisters on a red base. This blister group may itch, prickle, or burn. It can vary in size from that of a matchhead to a 25-cent piece or even larger. Although a cold sore can develop on any part of the body, it generally occurs on the mouth, the lips, or on the genital areas.

Up until a few years ago, doctors thought that cold sores of the

mouth and lips—transmitted by contact with infected saliva—
were invariably caused by a virus called herpesvirus Type 1. And
that cold sore-like infections below the waist—genital herpes—
were always caused by a closely-related organism, labeled herpesvirus Type 2. In recent years, however, due perhaps to our
changing mores and the growing popularity of oral sex, the Type 1
viruses can cause genital "cold sores" and the Type 2 herpesvirus
can cause mouth and lip lesions.

COLD SORES OF THE MOUTH AND LIPS

Whether you call them cold sores, fever blisters, or the medical
term herpes simplex, they all describe the same problem—a
problem that can literally lead to a pain in the neck.

Cold sores are caused by a virus. The primary, or initial,
infection with the herpes simplex virus usually occurs in early
childhood. The infection, however, may not cause any symptoms
for years while the virus lies dormant. Then suddenly, a variety of
factors can trigger an outbreak of blisters, the visible sign of the
infection. These factors include sun exposure, local injury (from
dental work, for example), emotional tension, colds and other
upper respiratory infections, various foods (chocolate, nuts, seafood), and, in rare instances, menstruation.

If left alone, the blisters rupture and form small ulcers. The
ulcers then form crusts and scabs and finally heal in ten to fourteen
days. As a rule, they do not leave scars.

If there is excessive pain or discomfort and the lymph glands
in the neck become swollen, it usually means that the virus has
caused a secondary infection. When this happens, you may need an
oral antibiotic.

We know of no single effective cure for cold sores and fever
blisters. Many over-the-counter remedies, however, are often effective in relieving the signs and symptoms of cold sores of the mouth
and lips.

If your cold sores are persistent or recurring, it is wise to
consult your dermatologist. In extreme cases, herpes simplex can
cause complications and lead to disease in the eyes, brain, and
internal organs.

GENITAL HERPES

Genital herpes, or cold sores of the genital area, is considered
a venereal disease because it is usually transmitted by sexual
contact. Affecting more than 500,000 Americans each year, genital

herpes is reportedly the most prevalent venereal disease among young Americans today, its incidence being greater than both gonorrhea and syphilis. It accounts for about 15 percent of all sexually transmitted diseases in this country.

The threat of genital herpes has become so widespread that many young, unmarried Americans have altered their sexual behavior to prevent contracting the disease. People are becoming more cautious about casual sex and thinking twice about the "one-night stand."

Like cold sores on the mouth and lips, genital herpes is transmitted by a virus. This virus is usually transmitted by direct sexual contact (genital to genital or mouth to genital) with a person who has an active herpes infection. There is even the risk of contracting the herpes virus from a towel or drinking cup or tester lipstick used by a person with open lesions. Given the opportunity, this virus can infect any portion of the body surface of a susceptible person. What is particularly disturbing are the unpredictable recurrences of these genital infections in the same person, at the same site, with a frequency that can be distressing, embarrassing and, at times, disabling. Fortunately, however, the herpes virus infections have a tendency to become milder with each recurrence.

How do you know if you have genital herpes? The average incubation period, that is, from the time of contact to when you first notice the symptoms, is roughly a week. Any number of signs and symptoms may precede or accompany a herpes infection of the genital region. These can include itching, mild burning and prickling sensations, pain during urination and sexual intercourse, fever, headache, and swollen lymph glands in the groin area.

Small groups of blisters commonly appear at the infected site, usually around the vagina or on the penis. These blisters break down in a few days leaving painful, shallow ulcers that, when not complicated by any other infection, heal in about a week to ten days.

For some people, a genital herpes infection is a painful, swollen inflammation. For others, the infection is relatively mild and transient, with few or no symptoms. People who are completely asymptomatic, and there are many, may act as reservoirs, or "carriers," for the disease, unknowingly affecting their sex partners. And so the question often posed by a spouse or a friend, "Who gave you (me) this herpes infection?" cannot be answered with any certainty.

If you develop a herpes infection a week after sex relations, you have not necessarily contracted herpes from your sex partner. The friction of intercourse may very well have activated a dormant herpes virus in your body.

And while the primary infection (meaning the first time one is afflicted with the condition) is acquired by direct sexual contact (genital to genital or mouth to genital), recurrences of genital herpes infections generally represent reactivation of a latent, hidden virus, rather than reinfection.

What causes these reactivations, these recurrences, and what are some of the triggering mechanisms? No one really knows.

After an active herpes episode, the virus retreats to and remains quietly hidden in a nerve root, thus making treatment difficult or impossible. After weeks, months, or even years, the virus, stirred up by any number of mechanisms, travels down the nerve path and reappears on the skin, starting up a new batch of small blisters with all the symptoms of the earlier herpes infection. Some of the reactivating mechanisms that have been implicated in provoking recurrences include mechanical injury, masturbation, sexual intercourse, fever, gastrointestinal upsets, sunburn, fatigue, overexertion, sleeplessness, poor nutrition, menstruation, psychic stress, and even sauna baths!

What is particularly disturbing about genital herpes is its serious consequences. Extensive herpes of the genital organs can cause excruciating pain during urination and sexual intercourse.

The consequences for pregnant women are especially grim. Genital herpes is three times more common in pregnant women than in nonpregnant women and results in a higher incidence of miscarriages and premature births.

Newborns who are infected during birth are unable to combat the virus with their immature immune systems. Thus, if an active genital herpes is present at the time of delivery, it can cause a devastating or fatal infection in the newborn as the infant passes through the birth canal. Therefore, most doctors recommend a Caesarean section for women who have an active herpes infection just before delivery.

In addition, women with genital herpes infections run a five times greater risk of cancer of the cervix. And for both women and men, there is a much higher incidence of other venereal infections, such as gonorrhea and syphilis.

There is a new test that takes just four hours to detect herpes simplex virus infections. This will help women avoid unnecessary Caesarean sections and it will help patients with herpes infections of the eye get prompt, often sight-saving, treatment.

While effective treatment for herpes is poor at best, you should consult your physician to try to prevent complications that could lead to severe secondary bacterial infection and spread of the disease.

Treatment of the active infection consists mainly of relieving the symptoms:

- Reduce the inflammation and swelling with warm baths or continuous compresses using cool, whole milk.
- Relieve the pain and itching with aspirin, antihistamines, and appropriate topical medications prescribed by your physician.
- Control any secondary bacterial and yeast infection, again with medications prescribed by your doctor.
- Since urine can cause excruciating pain and stinging of vulvar lesions in women, protect those delicate areas with zinc oxide paste.

As far as specific treatments for herpes, there are as many different kinds as there are doctors. Everything works—and nothing works.

Past and present treatments have included applying cortisone-like antibiotic creams and ointments, ice cubes, ether, nail polish remover, liquid nitrogen, cortisone-type sprays, and a dozen different other topical (surface) medications. None of these treatments has yet withstood the test of time, but many doctors will still swear by their particular method.

One theory suggests that oral contraceptives help to prevent recurrences. Women taking the birth control pills report fewer recurrences than women who do not. There is also some evidence that the chemicals in most contraceptive foams have an antiviral effect on the genital herpes virus.

The only proven treatment for genital herpes, and the only one that Food and Drug Administration has cleared, is acyclovir, a prescription capsule that goes under the trade name of *Zovirax*. Acyclovir, the first antiviral agent to be effective against genital herpes, is *not* a cure, and there is no proof that it prevents the spread of genital herpes. But it does relieve the symptoms, it reduces the shedding of the virus, and it shortens the duration of an attack. If taken for at least six months, three capsules a day *may* reduce the frequency and the severity of recurrent episodes of genital herpes.

Also sold as an ointment, acyclovir will usually alleviate the symptoms of burning and itching and help speed up the healing process for an initial episode of genital herpes.

Unfortunately, we cannot eradicate the virus by simply treating the local infection. For those of you who have genital herpes, I leave you with this sobering thought: you have it for life. And every time it recurs, it can potentially infect other people.

Here are a few suggestions, however, to prevent spread of the disease:

- Practice good genital hygiene. That means "soap and water."
- Wear loose, soft, cotton clothing and avoid rubbing and chafing.
- If you're uncircumcised and have recurrent genital herpes, I recommend circumcision.
- When you have oral or genital lesions, don't have sex.
- Use a barrier method of contraception (condoms, spermicidal jellies, contraceptive foams, and diaphragm) if you are unsure whether you or your partner are actively infected.

The cure for these herpes infections will ultimately come when someone discovers an antiviral antibiotic that will destroy the virus in its dormant lair, the nerve root. And, if we are able to produce a safe vaccine such as those given to children in a single dose, herpes, like polio, smallpox, influenza, typhoid, and diphtheria, will forever be eradicated.

We're working on it.

For further information about herpes, write to:

American Social Health Association (ASHA)
100 Capitola Drive, Suite 200
Box 13827
Research Triangle Park, NC 27709
Ms Cyndi Spinden, Business Manager
919/361– 2742

TREATING COLD SORES

Before a cold sore blister appears, there may be a tingling and itching sensation of the affected part. To help reduce the size of the cold sore that's sure to show up, apply an ice cube to the area for about five minutes every half hour or so.

There are many over-the-counter cold sore preparations that may help if applied early enough. Try either of the following:

Campho-Phenique Liquid or *Gel* (Winthrop)

Blistex Medicated Lip Ointment (Blistex)

Follow the directions on the label of each container.

If your cold sores show up when you're exposed to the sun, use a sunscreen lip balm such as *PreSun Lip Protector* (Westwood) and take two aspirins a couple of hours before you go out in the sun.

SHINGLES

"In Jerusalem, it was reported that Premier Golda Meir is over the worst of her shingles attack she suffered three weeks ago, but still has an irritating rash on her midriff. Doctors from as far away as California and Italy have offered diagnostic consultation to Mrs. Meir's physician and, according to the Jerusalem Post, sympathizers have been sending her medical advice and remedies for shingles through many Israeli embassies abroad."

New York Times, January 24, 1975.

Shingles is an inflammation of a nerve which causes pain, itching, a rash, or all three. It affects an estimated 300,000 people in the United States each year.

The word *shingles* comes from the Latin *cingulus* meaning a girdle. It has been known from biblical times as the creeping eruption that girdles the body.

Shingles has nothing to do with "nerves" in the emotional sense. You might hear someone say, "Oh! She's a nervous wreck. That's why she came down with the shingles." Nonsense. Because shingles affects a *nerve*, many people mistake this to mean that it is a nervous condition.

The condition has affected its share of celebrities—Golda Meir, Arthur Rubinstein, and former President Nixon immediately come to mind—and that notoriety also has led to many misconceptions about it.

Shingles, the technical name for which is herpes zoster, is caused by a virus. It's the same virus that's responsible for chicken pox; it actually represents a reactivation of latent chicken pox viruses from an earlier infection.

Like chicken pox, shingles is usually a once-in-a-lifetime condition. Unlike chicken pox, however, it is only slightly contagious.

Although shingles can affect any age group, it's more prevalent and more painful in older people. And since shingles can attack any nerve, no area of the body surface is immune. Depending upon the severity of the pain and the location of the nerve involved, one can mistake shingles in its early stages for attacks of appendicitis, kidney stones, gallbladder trouble, pleurisy, and even facial neuralgia and toothache.

The virus of shingles attacks a nerve root in the brain or spinal cord and follows the course of that nerve only. Early symptoms include a feeling of fatigue, headache, a slight fever, and a mild drawing pain over the involved area. The pain characteristically involves only one side.

The infected areas of the skin become red and itchy, and a rash, made up of small blisters, often follows, usually in groups, along the path of the affected nerve. These blisters last for about two weeks and then rupture, forming crusts.

Because each nerve extends to a very specific part of the body on either the left or right side, the blisters usually have a ribbon-like or branching configuration, forming a semicircle on one side of the body.

In children and young adults, shingles usually runs a mild and quick course, and the average sufferer will recover without any therapy. In older people, however, the pain may be excruciating, the itching may be intense, and the blisters may become crusted and infected.

Complications can arise from even the mildest form of shingles, so it is important that a physician examine any suspected case. Your doctor can prescribe various internal medications, such as antibiotics, cortisone-like drugs, analgesics and antihistamines, to relieve the pain, itching and inflammation, as well as soothing salves and ointments to relieve the dermatitis and possibly prevent spread of the disease.

When shingles involves the eye, you should consult an ophthalmologist (a physician who specializes in diseases of the eye) to prevent severe damage to the cornea. Arthur Rubinstein, one of the country's greatest pianists, had to retire from the concert stage in 1976, when an attack of shingles left him nearly blind.

Other complications of shingles which may occur are scarring where the blisters had been, extreme fatigue and malaise during the period of recovery, and persistent dull or severe pain (postherpetic neuralgia) which may linger for months or longer after the rash has disappeared.

Occurring in more than half the patients over the age of fifty, this oftentimes exquisite pain that follows an episode of herpes zoster, can be extremely disabling. A variety of attempts to control or reduce this relentless torment has met with variable success. A new topical medication, capsaicin, holds some promise in relieving some of this distressing symptom. This over-the-counter product, called *Zostrix*, should be applied three or four times a day, with relief of the pain anticipated in about two or three weeks. It should be continued for a period of several months, and for those who have been suffering from chronic pain, treatment over several years should be expected.

While there are no cures, as such, for shingles, many dermatologists have been prescribing acyclovir (*Zovirax*) orally in large doses in an attempt to shorten the course of the disease and, possibly, to diminish some of the complications.

There are no measures known to prevent shingles. You may save yourself some worry, however, by avoiding direct contact with someone who has shingles. If you are older, and therefore more susceptible to shingles, you should also avoid young children who have chicken pox. Doctors will sometimes prescribe injections of gamma globulin for patients who are otherwise very ill and who have been exposed to persons who have either chicken pox or shingles.

If you do have shingles—some dermatologists call this "second-time" chicken pox—refrain from contact with infants and children who have never had chicken pox, and avoid people who are undergoing chemotherapy.

Shingles almost always limits itself to one side of the body. So, if you have a rash on both sides, chances are that shingles is not the culprit.

TREATING SHINGLES

For the early, blistery rash, use soothing compresses to help relieve the inflammation, control the itching, and dry up the blisters. Follow the directions for applying compresses on page 217, using the following:

Bluboro Powder (Herbert)
Directions for use are on the package.

After using the compresses, and when the blisters have begun to dry up, use any of the following anti-itch medications whenever necessary:

Hytone Cream 0.5% (Dermik)

Sarna Lotion (Stiefel)

Schamberg's Lotion (C&M Pharmacal)

Directions for use are on the containers.

If the itching persists, take either of the following antihistamines every 4 hours as necessary.

Chlor-Trimeton Tablets [4 mg] (Schering)

Dimetane Tablets [4 mg] (Robins)

See directions and cautions on the labels for proper dosage.

For accompanying pain, take any pain-reliever (aspirin, Tylenol, Anacin, etc.) in appropriate doses.

For the severe pain of postherpetic neuralgia, try the new, over-the-counter cream, *Zostrix (GenDerm)*, and use according to directions on the package.

Note: If your shingles has any of the following characteristics, see your dermatologist:

- Occurs around the eye or on the tip of the nose
- Is widespread
- Appears infected
- Is extremely painful or itchy, or
- Has not responded to the treatment outlined above.

IMPETIGO

Impetigo is a highly contagious, unsightly skin infection caused by the streptococcus and staphylococcus bacteria. The medical term for this condition, appropriately, is impetigo contagiosa.

Impetigo appears as thick, stuck on, honey-colored crusts usually around the nostrils and mouth, although any portion of the skin surface may be affected. It occurs primarily in children, but adults can fall victim, too, usually by direct contact with infected children.

Impetigo begins on damaged skin, when the outer protective layers are injured and the normal resistance of the skin is lowered. This damage can be a result of cuts, bruises, insect bites, or other skin diseases, such as chicken pox, cold sores, or acne. Healthy skin seems to act as a barrier to suppress these harmful bacteria.

The mouth and nose, which suffer constant rubbing and wiping, are the prime areas on which impetigo begins. The infectious germs are carried to other parts of the body by dirty fingers and fingernails and by unclean towels, utensils, and clothing. These germs can also spread to other people who have direct contact with infected persons, especially through kissing, wrestling, or other such contact sports.

Once impetigo takes hold, it spreads very easily, even to normal healthy skin, and may last for several weeks. If not controlled, it can lead to internal infections accompanied by fever, fatigue, and swollen lymph glands.

Those infected with impetigo should seek prompt medical attention. A doctor's care can help prevent generalized spread, especially to other members of the family and friends, and possibly prevent the serious internal complications that may arise, such as kidney infections.

Treatment consists of gently removing the crusts and thoroughly cleansing the affected areas four times daily with a good antibacterial soap, such as Dial or Safeguard. If the crusts stick stubbornly to the underlying skin, you may need to apply warm water compresses to lift them off.

After each thorough washing, rub an antibiotic ointment into the affected areas. *Do not cover the area with bandages or gauze.* Exposure to air will help kill many types of germs and speed the healing process.

If the condition is extensive and severe, your physician may prescribe an oral antibiotic, such as penicillin or erythromycin, or a penicillin injection.

The following are some additional measures that help eliminate impetigo and prevent its spread:

- Wash hands thoroughly and frequently with an antibacterial soap.
- Avoid touching sores because infection can spread easily to other parts of your body.
- Keep fingernails trimmed and scrupulously clean at all times.
- Change your towels daily.
- Since impetigo is contagious, avoid close contact with friends and relatives, and keep the children home during the acute, crusted stage of the disease.

- Continue treatment for seven to ten days after all the crusts are gone.

If the lesions persist after several days of therapy, contact your doctor for further treatment. This treatment may include an oral antibiotic or a penicillin injection.

TREATING IMPETIGO

In the superficial variety of impetigo, seen on the face and caused mainly by staphylococcal organisms, many physicians believe that thorough cleansing and appropriate topical therapy, without oral or injectable antibiotics, can do the trick.

Wash the affected areas thoroughly 3 or 4 times daily with any of the following:

Dial Soap (Armour)
Safeguard Soap (Procter & Gamble)
Shield (Lever Brothers)

After washing thoroughly, gently remove any *loosely* attached crusts. This is best done with clean, washed tweezers. Then apply one of the following antibacterial ointments 3 times daily:

Mycitracin Ointment (Upjohn)
Polysporin Ointment (Burroughs Wellcome)

Continue the washing and ointment applications for at least a week after the crusts have disappeared. If the lesions persist despite this treatment, see your dermatologist.

Note: Some doctors recommend internal antibiotics for the treatment of impetigo to prevent some of the rare complications, such as kidney infections.

INSECT BITES & STINGS

Spring and summer mean lush foliage, sunshine, flowers and—The Sting.

If you work or play in fields and gardens, bees, wasps, hornets, and yellow jackets buzz around loaded with nuisance, pain, and sometimes danger.

Bites and stings, for the most part, are only an annoyance and rarely cause more than slight, temporary discomfort. The reactions to insect stings are caused by either allergic mechanisms or sensitivity to certain chemicals, toxins, or enzymes in the venom. Occasionally, these reactions can be fatal in sensitive individuals.

Insect sting allergy has been recognized since antiquity. Hiero-glyphics on the wall of the tomb of King Menes in Egypt record his death, in 2621 BC, from a wasp or hornet sting. And today, there are more deaths in the United States from insect stings than from snakebites.

The honeybee and yellow jacket are responsible for most stings. Although they may similar appearances, these two insects have very different habits. The honeybee is a social insect that uses a stinger to inject venom into its victim. A yellow jacket is a wasp that can both bite and sting. The honeybee usually does not sting unless disturbed, but when sufficiently provoked to attack, it leaves its barbed stinger and attached venom sac in the skin of its victim.

The simple, normal sting, the one you are most likely to encounter, causes varying degrees of pain at the site of the sting lasting for a few minutes. Redness, swelling, and itching of the area follow. If no complications arise, all traces of the sting will usually disappear within a few hours.

In the exaggerated type of local reaction, there is more itching and swelling. The symptoms may last longer, and there may be a great deal of discomfort.

The treatment for most insect bites and stings is the same. In the case of a bee sting, however, you must remove the barbed stinger and attached venom sac as quickly as possible, as the walls of the sac contract and continue to inject venom.

Never try to pull the stinger out or squeeze the area in which the stinger is embedded. This will break the venom sac, releasing more of the toxic or allergic substances and aggravating your symptoms. Instead, gently scrape the area with a knife blade or fingernail until the stinger and sac have been dislodged.

After you remove the stinger and venom sac, follow these steps to treat the simple insect sting:

- Wash the area with soap and water.
- Use ice packs or cold compresses for 30 to 45 minutes to reduce the inflammation and swelling.
- Apply a paste made up of one teaspoonful of unseasoned meat tenderizer and water. This often results in prompt, lasting relief.
- Treat any hives and itching by applying phenolated ca-lamine lotion every 3 or 4 hours.
- If severe swelling, itching, and pain persist, call your doctor.

You may need an antihistamine or cortisone-like drug to counteract the bee venom.
- If you are stung on your foot or leg, elevate it and keep it at rest.

Insects are somewhat discriminating, so follow these steps to make yourself less of a target for bites and stings.

- Always wear shoes outside. Bare feet are the most vulnerable areas for insect attacks. (Bees love clover and yellow jackets live in the ground.)
- Avoid scented soaps, perfumes, colognes, hair sprays, and other scented products. These odors attract insects.
- Wear light-colored, smooth fabrics. Bright, flowery prints and dark, rough clothing attract insects as well.
- Avoid bright jewelry and other metal objects. Again, insects find these very alluring.
- If you come into contact with a stinging insect, avoid sudden and dramatic motions. Move away very slowly and do not flap, wave, or swat.
- Avoid touching insect nests.
- Keep house screens in good repair.
- Keep garbage cans covered at all times.
- Be especially alert after rain; pollen is scarce and insects become more easily excited.

A word on insect repellents: Insect repellents are not insecticides. They do not kill mosquitos, ticks, chiggers, fleas, or the many varieties of biting flies. They just discourage them from biting you. And they do not work against stinging insects like bees, wasps, or ants.

To prevent against mosquito and fly bites, use insect repellents on exposed parts of your body and on your clothing. Do not use repellents on broken skin and be particularly careful when applying them on children. Pregnant women should not use them at any time. And since the active ingredient is flammable, do not apply them near fires.

TREATING BITES & STINGS

For a few, localized insect bites, where there is redness, swelling, and itching, the best immediate treatment is applying ice. An ice cube, held on the bite areas for 5 to 10 minutes, will usually give prompt relief of the pain, itching, and swelling.

Another good "home remedy" is the application of a paste made up of one teaspoonful of unseasoned meat tenderizer and a few drops of water. Applying this to the bite or sting may provide immediate relief.

Other preparations that can give relief of the itching associated with insect bites include the following:

Hytone Cream 0.5% (Dermik)
Sarna Lotion (Stiefel)
Campho-Phenique Liquid or *Gel* (Winthrop)
Directions for use are on the labels.

To relieve prolonged itching of insect bites, take either of the following antihistamines every 3 or 4 hours.

Chlor-Trimeton Tablets [4 mg] (Schering)
Dimetane Tablets [4 mg] (Robins)
See directions and cautions on the labels for proper dosage.

If none of the above remedies relieves your symptoms, call your doctor.

INFESTATIONS

While parasites are not considered a major problem for people in the United States, there are two types of similar organisms which recently have caused virtual epidemics. These organisms, called ectoparasites, are lice and mites.

Infestations with lice (true insects) and mites (insect-like organisms) cause intensely itchy, annoying skin problems. Unless diagnosed and treated properly, these conditions can persist and eventually spread to family members, classmates, and friends.

LICE

Lice are small, wingless insects about one-eighth of an inch in length. They have been around for centuries and have flourished on both the rich and poor.

Associated with wars and disease in the Middle Ages, lice carry typhus, a disease which has been known to wipe out entire armies. They were extremely prevalent throughout the world until World War II, when DDT almost eradicated this annoying and dread pestilence. However, the recent ban on DDT as a hazardous substance, along with the increase in social contact and world travel, has contributed to a resurgence of louse infestation. Today lice have become a major public health problem throughout the world. Aggravated by poor living conditions, lack of personal cleanliness, and overcrowding, this infestation has reached epidemic proportions. Lice are so common in Japan that pediculicides are distributed free in Japanese bathhouses.

The main symptoms of louse infestation, known technically as pediculosis, is a relentless, maddening itch caused by the saliva of the female louse.

There are three kinds of lice affecting three different body areas: head lice, pubic lice, and body lice. Although each type has a different shape, they all feed by biting the skin and sucking the blood.

The adult female louse lays eggs (nits) which she firmly attaches with a glue-like substance to hairs or to fibers of clothing. The eggs hatch in about ten days and reach maturity in about two weeks. Lice have a life span of about one month.

HEAD LICE

Head lice have become especially prevalent in recent years, particularly among school children in urban areas. They make their home in your hair, causing intense itching on your scalp, the back of your neck, and behind your ears, and, in severe cases, swollen lymph glands in your neck. For some reason, head lice are almost never seen in blacks.

If you look closely, you can see the small, silvery egg cases attached to individual hair shafts. Usually these nits will be close to the scalp, no more than a half-inch from where the hair begins. Although they resemble dandruff, they are much more difficult to remove than dandruff flakes because of the sticky, cement-like substance the female louse secretes to attach the nits.

Head lice are transmitted by direct contact, by personal items such as combs, brushes, and pillowcases, and through clothing such as hats, scarves, ribbons, and other head coverings. If one person in a family or classroom has head lice, there is a good possibility that others in the same home or class will have it, too.

If you have head lice, treatment is relatively simple and very effective. *Kwell*, a prescription shampoo will cure a case of head lice in five minutes. One shampoo for five minutes. That's it! There are also non-prescription shampoos (see treatment section below) that work about as well.

After shampooing, you may still see eggs attached to the hair shafts, but these are now dead. To get rid of the unsightly but harmless dead nits, apply dilute vinegar (one-half vinegar and one-half water) to your scalp to loosen them and then back comb with a fine-tooth comb.

To prevent the spread of lice, thoroughly wash all articles of clothing that are suspected of having nits or adult lice.

PUBIC LICE ("CRAB" LICE)

Pubic lice infestation, called "crabs," is a highly contagious sexually-transmitted diseases. There has been a steady increase in its incidence, with about 2 million new cases in 1984 alone. For some reason, "crabs" are more common in females between the ages of 15 and 19, and more common in males over the age of 20.

Usually you get pubic lice through sexual or other close physical contact, but they are also transmitted by just sharing a bed or wearing the clothes of an infested person, and even, rarely, from toilet seats!

The usual symptom of pubic lice is a maddening itch (especially at night), that scratching doesn't relieve. Like head lice, the nits of pubic lice are usually glued in clusters to the short hair shafts and resemble the flakes of dandruff. Crabs usually set up housekeeping in the pubic region, but during warm, dark, and quiet periods, the adult lice, along with their eggs, migrate to other short-haired areas of the body—the bellybutton, chest, beard, and mustache in men, the armpits, and even the eyelashes.

The treatment for pubic lice is essentially the same as that for head lice (see treatment section below). For lice and nits that have found their way to your eyelashes, apply *Johnson's Baby Shampoo* with a *Q-Tip* two or three times daily. This should cure the condition in a few days.

BODY LICE

Infestation with body lice is not very common in the United States. Unlike head and crab lice, body lice bite the skin but live in the seams of clothing. Treat the clothing, and the rash will disappear.

SCABIES

Scabies is a common and contagious skin disease. Like lice, it has reached epidemic proportions in the United States. Although scabies is often associated with poverty and its crowded living conditions and poor hygiene, there has been a definite increase of the disease among the more affluent. Anybody and everybody can have scabies.

Scabies is caused by a mite, a tiny creature, mistakenly

referred to as an insect. This mite measures about one seventy-fifth of an inch in length, so small that it is barely visible to the naked eye. The mites burrow into the skin and spread from one individual to the next through personal and sexual contact. Animals, primarily dogs, carry a different form of scabies which they can pass on to humans to cause a similar condition.

Scabies is characterized by intense itching, due to an allergy to the female mite and the eggs and feces she deposits underneath the upper layers of the skin. This itching becomes more intense at night, when the tiny organisms become more active, or when the person gets overheated or removes his or her clothing. Often the itching is so severe that it leads to nervousness and loss of sleep. And since the scratching often causes bleeding, an infested person may have bloodied sheets, pajamas, or underwear.

The scabies mite is most fond of attacking the webs of the fingers, the inner surfaces of the wrists, and the elbows. Other common areas where the mites set up housekeeping are the chest near the armpits, the area around the bellybutton, the buttocks, the nipples, and the penis. As a rule, infestations above the neck are extremely rare, except in infants and young children.

Because scabies mimics several other itchy skin conditions, it often goes undiagnosed or misdiagnosed. Various salves and lotions may alleviate your itching for a short period of time, but if scabies is the culprit, the mites will thrive and often cause secondary infection requiring antibiotic therapy.

Once the proper diagnosis has been established—and only a physician is capable of recognizing it—the cure is relatively simple. *Kwell Lotion*, a prescription medication, will cure almost all cases of scabies with only one or two applications. (Do not use *Kwell Lotion* more than twice and do not use it on children under the age of six.) In addition, wash or dry clean all contaminated clothing and linens. And, since scabies spreads so easily, it is vitally important that every person in the household and all sex partners of the person affected should be treated whether or not they have any symptoms.

So if you have persistent, widespread itching that occurs below the neck, that is more pronounced at night, and that is unrelieved by the usual simple baths and lotions, see your dermatologist. Fortunately, the nasty scabies mite succumbs to a swift and simple cure.

TREATING LICE
The following are a couple of good, over-the-counter treatments for head lice:

Rid (Leeming)

A-200 Pyrinate (Norcliff Thayer)

Directions for use are on the labels.

To restore body and luster to hair following scalp applications, follow with a mild shampoo.

If necessary, you can repeat this treatment, but do not exceed two applications within twenty four hours.

To prevent reinfestation with lice, thoroughly wash all articles of clothing that are suspected of having nits or adult lice.

TREATING SCABIES
There are no over-the-counter remedies for scabies. If you suspect that you or members of your family have scabies, or if you have had any recent contact with someone who had scabies, see your dermatologist. He or she can make the diagnosis and prescribe the appropriate medication.

HIVES

Hives is a very common disorder. At least 20% of the general population will develop some form of hive-like eruption in the course of a lifetime.

What are hives? Contrary to popular opinion, it is *not* a disease. Caused by the release of a chemical called histamine, hives— physicians call it urticaria—is a symptom of some disorder or allergic mechanism going on in the body. Hives appear on the skin and mucous membranes in the form of itching, stinging, and burning wheals (welts), surrounded by a zone of redness. They resemble big mosquito bites. Hives come in a variety of sizes and shapes and can appear just about anywhere on your body, but mostly on pressure points—where you sit or lean.

When the wheals are very large and the loose tissue of the eyelids, lips and tongue swell up to form actual disfigurement, the condition is called angioedema, or "bull hives." Hives may involve the mucous membranes of the mouth and throat, and in rare cases may even obstruct breathing so severely that one requires heroic medical methods to prevent suffocation.

Like coughing or sneezing, which may signal a response to an upper respiratory infection or hay fever, hives are a clue which alerts us to abnormal goings-on in our system. For example, it may be a response to an infection, an allergic reaction to some strange food or drug, or the result of emotional tension.

It is extremely difficult to pinpoint the specific cause of a case of hives, mainly because the possibilities are endless. In the acute type of hives, where the itching and wheals appear quickly and fade in a few minutes or hours, it is somewhat easier to uncover the culprit: a strange food, an emotional upset, a penicillin injection, a new medication, or some recent infection such as chicken pox, mononucleosis, or an upper respiratory ailment. Unfortunately, in the chronic form, which occurs most commonly in middle-aged women, and which may last for months or even years, the culprit is much more difficult to determine.

The most common causes of hives are certain foods and drugs. Strawberries, nuts, chocolate, fish and shellfish, milk, eggs, pork, oranges, bananas, and many other edibles, such as the artificial sweetener aspartame, can cause hives.

Of the various drugs and medications, penicillin is probably the most common cause. If you are allergic to penicillin and suffer from hives, you should avoid milk and certain cheeses, such as blue cheese and Roquefort. Milk and other dairy products may contain enough penicillin to prolong hives for years. A woman who is allergic to penicillin may develop hives after having intercourse with a man who has been taking the drug. This phenomenon occurs because penicillin levels in semen can be as high as those in the blood, causing the allergic reaction. The systematic use of other antibiotics, such as tetracycline, in cattle feed also can cause hives.

Another common cause is aspirin. When you realize that Americans consume more than 15 million pounds of aspirin each year, it's little wonder that we see so many reactions from it.

Related to aspirin are other hive-producing chemicals known as salicylates. Salicylates appear in such products as root beer, wintergreen and mint flavorings, commercial bakery products, and mixes. Certain food dyes and preservatives (such as sodium benzoate), insulin, and various vaccines to protect against measles and polio may also be common offenders. So is menthol, found in such diverse products as cigarettes, toothpastes, candies, jellies, Noxzema, room deodorants, lozenges, and shaving creams.

Some people get hives from inhaling substances such as

animal dander (from cats, dogs, or horses), house dust, pollen, molds, certain plants, and flour in bakeries. Others break out in hives when they touch something cold or when they touch something hot, and still others, when they are exposed to sunlight. Some even get hives when pressure is applied to their skin, as in the shower.

There are certain types of hives which are of psychogenic origin. Fear, anger, and stress are the primary psychological factors responsible.

Underlying infections of the teeth, sinuses, gastrointestinal, respiratory, and genitourinary tracts all can cause hives. Hives is also associated with viral diseases such as hepatitis and infectious mononucleosis.

The treatment of hives consists of identifying and eliminating the cause of the condition. You—the patient—must be the detective. What food did you eat? What medication did you take? Anything new? Anything different? Have you been in some strange place? What different inhalants or sprays have you been exposed to lately? Any recent emotional tensions?

See your doctor if your hives are persistent, recurring, or severe. It is important that you provide as much information as you can to your physician. Only a physician can unearth the orgin and nature of your hives, and only a physician can eradicate them. You may need a thorough physical examination, blood tests, X-rays, allergy testing, and other laboratory analyses to rule out any internal infection such as hepatitis.

For acute, temporary hives, over-the-counter antihistamines taken orally usually relieve the symptoms promptly, at least until your next exposure to the culprit. If these don't work, prescription medications, such as *Seldane*, *Atarax*, or *Hismanal* might do the job.

Finding the cause of chronic, recurrent hives is often a difficult, frustrating, and lengthy process, and requires patience and extensive detective work. Only when you are able to discover the cause, can you prevent your hives from recurring.

TREATING HIVES

Until you've identified and eliminated the culprit that's causing your hives, you can try to ease its annoying symptoms.

To soothe the itching of generalized hives, take lukewarm baths in either of the following bath oils:

Alpha Keri Shower and Bath Oil (Westwood)

Nutraderm Bath Oil (Owen)
Directions for use are on the labels.
Apply any of the following anti-itch preparations every three or four hours:
  Hytone Cream 0.5% (Dermik)
  Schamberg's Lotion (C&M Pharmacal)
  Sarna Lotion (Stiefel)
  Directions for use are on the labels.
If you need extra relief from itching, try either of the following antihistamines:
  Chlor-Trimeton [4 mg] (Schering)
  Dimetane [4 mg] (Robins)
  Directions for use and cautions are on the labels.

PITYRIASIS ROSEA

Pityriasis rosea is a most perplexing skin ailment. No one knows what causes it or what makes it disappear in a matter of weeks. We *do* know that it is usually a mild condition and that it is probably not contagious, even though small epidemics of the disease have occurred in Turkish baths, military establishments, and fraternity houses. If it is contagious, no one has been able to discover the germ that might be responsible.

Pityriasis rosea-like rashs can also occur in people taking various medications: penicillin, Accutane, Flagyl, barbiturates, beta-blockers, and others.

Commonly mistaken for ringworm, pityriasis rosea is a unique disorder. It usually begins as a single, large, round or oval pinkish patch, known as the "mother" or "herald" patch. The most common sites for this solitary lesion are the chest, the back, or the abdomen. This is followed in about two weeks by a blossoming of small, flat, oval, scaly patches of similar color usually distributed in a Christmas tree pattern over the chest and back.

This eruption seldom itches and usually limits itself to areas from the neck to the knees. It is more common in adolescents and young adults and in the spring and autumn. It disappears as mysteriously as it came, the older lesions fading first, in about six to eight weeks, without leaving any marks or scars and without causing any complications. It rarely crops up in the same family at the same time, it is not a sign of ill health, and it doesn't affect unborn children of pregnant women who are afflicted with it. And, it almost never recurs.

In other words, it's a pretty friendly skin condition!

There are, of course, exceptions, as there are in most skin diseases. For example, the herald plaque, which is supposed to signal the coming of a batch of smaller lesions, may be neither large nor conspicuous. Also, while the normal rash, at its peak, follows the Christmas tree pattern, it may cover the entire body. Occasionally, the condition may be accompanied by fierce and uncontrollable itching, and, even more rarely, by fever, malaise, loss of appetite, and swollen lymph glands in the neck.

I have seen pityriasis rosea last for over three months, and I have seen cases in the summer and winter. Several of my patients have been young children with intensely itchy "bumps" on not only the trunk but the entire face and scalp, and I've even noted recurrences of this condition time and again. But, fortunately, these are only the exceptions. Usually, it is an extremely mild condition.

The treatment of pityriasis rosea is purely symptomatic: if it doesn't itch, leave it alone. If your itching is mild, soothing baths and a hydrocortisone cream or lotion applied two or three times daily should give you adequate relief. However, if the itching becomes intense and the rash begins to spread very rapidly, you should consult a dermatologist. He or she will prescribe appropriate oral medication and sometimes ultraviolet light treatments to relieve the itching and shorten the course of the disease.

One bit of advice: for your own peace of mind, don't take too much stock in nonprofessional opinions. Some people, seeing the sudden onset and spread of this strange rash, have shown it to relatives, friends, and the friendly pharmacist, who tell them that they probably have either ringworm, syphilis, AIDS, or some bizarre blood disorder. The most important consideration for those with pityriasis rosea is the reassurance that it is neither serious, contagious, infectious, nor malignant, and that it will eventually disappear in a matter of a few weeks without leaving permanent marks or scars.

TREATING PITYRIASIS ROSEA

Since pityriasis rosea is usually fairly widespread, the best method of treating it is with soothing baths. For the scaling and itching that accompany it, use either:

Alpha Keri Bath Oil (Westwood) or

Nutraderm Bath Oil (Owen)

Directions for use are on each container.

For localized itching, apply any of the following to the affected areas 2 or 3 times daily:

Hytone Cream 0.5% (Dermik)

Sarna Lotion (Stiefel)

Schamberg's Lotion (C&M Pharmacal)

Directions for use are on the labels.

For the dryness that remains after the condition has run its course, use any of the following:

Keri Lotion (Westwood)

Nutraderm Lotion (Owen)

Sofenol 5 (C&M Pharmacal)

Directions for use are on the labels.

If itching persists, take either of the following antihistamines:

Chlor-Trimeton [4 mg] (Schering)

Dimetane [4 mg] (Robins)

Directions for use and cautions are on the labels.

ALLERGY RASHES

More and more, people of all ages and from all walks of life are exposed to thousands of different substances which can affect the skin through their use at home, work, or play. The enormous increase in the number of new chemical-containing products found in industry and in the marketplace has been responsible for a large percentage of skin eruptions called contact dermatitis.

What do we mean by contact dermatitis? Simply stated, a contact dermatitis is a redness or inflammation of the skin which results from actual contact with a variety of natural or manufactured materials. Where and how much the inflammation shows up depend on where the troublesome material touched the skin.

The different types of contact dermatitis fall under two categories: reactions due to irritation and reactions due to allergy.

REACTIONS DUE TO IRRITATION (Primary Irritants)

A primary irritant is a substance strong enough to cause a demonstrable reaction and actual physical damage to the skin, in a high percentage of people, following initial exposure. The inflammation it causes may manifest itself merely as redness, or it may be severe enough to cause blistering and ulcers. It is similar in appearance to a mechanical injury or burn. Skin and deeper tissues are damaged, followed by inflammation and occasional scarring. How quickly the reaction occurs and how severe it is will depend upon the type of irritant, its concentration, the length of exposure time, and the extent of contact.

Examples of strong primary irritants are lye, nitric acid, gasoline, turpentine, paint remover, and chemicals used for hair straightening. These require only a few hours, or even minutes, in some cases, to damage the skin. And they affect almost everybody. Mild irritants—soaps, solvents, laundry bleaches, and metal cleansers—affect a smaller percentage of people and may require several days of contact to produce an effect.

Irritations due to chemicals are treated like burns. The goal is to soothe, comfort, and prevent infection and scarring.

REACTIONS DUE TO ALLERGY (Hypersensitivity)

In simple medical terms, an allergy develops when your body overreacts to a foreign substance. The reaction can take place in various parts of the body. In your respiratory system, it can show up as hay fever or asthma. In your intestinal tract, it may manifest itself as stomach cramps or pains. And in your nervous system, it can result in migraine headaches. On the skin, it often takes the form of redness, itching, swelling, and sometimes blistering. Why a person becomes sensitized to a material is not clear, but it appears to involve the person's immune system.

Just about one out of every ten patients who see a doctor for some skin problem will find out that he or she has an "allergic contact dermatitis." Unlike the primary irritant dermatitis, allergic contact dermatitis requires a few days to a week before the symptoms appear.

We can't predict who will and who won't have an allergic reaction. Sometimes, a person could be touching the same material over and over again for many years without anything happening. Then suddenly he or she breaks out in a rash. Some people have allergies to a lot of different products they use everyday, while others use the very same products and never develop any signs of allergy. No one knows why.

There are myriad substances that we come in contact with all the time that could cause an allergic reaction, no matter how healthy we are. To find out just what the culprit is takes some good detective work. The majority of these substances are found in the home or marketplace. The following are some likely places to start the search:

CLOTHING
- Wool, silk, furs, synthetic fibers, gloves, stockings, and underwear elastic.
- Clothing additives and finishes used to improve the look and feel of clothing—"wash and wear," permanent press, and antishrinkage and softening chemicals, especially the perfumed fabric softeners used in clothes dryers, such as Bounce and Cling-Free.
- Dyes—particularly the dark brown, dark blue, and black.
- Rubber materials, adhesives, chemicals used to tan leather, and shoe dyes. (A dermatitis on the top of the feet and toes is almost always due to an allergy to something in your footwear and not athlete's foot.)
- Leather goods, such as handbags, gloves, and wallets.
- Parts of clothing and jewelry containing nickel, including rings, necklaces, earrings, bra clasps, zippers, snaps, hairpins, and metal eyeglass frames.

HOUSEHOLD ITEMS
- Glues, paints and varnishes, waxes and polishes, oil stains, plastics, soaps, detergents, and household cleansers.

FOODS
- Certain vegetables, fruit juices, and various spices.

PLANTS
- Poison ivy, hyacinth, tulips, ragweed.

CHEMICALS
- Pesticides, insecticides, and fertilizers.

OVER-THE-COUNTER DRUGS
- Poison ivy remedies containing benzocaine and zironium.
- Athlete's foot medications.
- Hair removal products for legs, underarms, and bikini areas.
- Analgesic balms and liniments for burns, sunburn, and pain.
- Depilatory agents.
- Tar preparations for psoriasis and eczema.
- Acne lotions, scrubs, and gels.
- And hundreds of others.

If you take a look at where a rash appears, you can usually figure out what might be the cause. For example, if the rash is on your face, you should suspect cosmetics, nose drops, sprays, eyeglass frames, and over-the-counter lotions, creams, and ointments. On the earlobes, consider earrings containing nickel (almost all do), hair dyes and sprays, perfumes, and other scented lotions. A rash on the neck can be caused by necklaces, hair dyes and sprays, collars, and scarves. In the armpits, consider antiperspirants and deodorants.

For contact dermatitis of your legs and feet, think of socks, stockings, pants, and shoes, as well as plants such as poison ivy.

Irritation in the genital or anal area could be caused by colored or perfumed toilet paper, jock itch medication, feminine hygiene sprays, scented tampons, pads and panty liners, douches, hemorrhoid treatments, suppositories, and birth control creams and devices.

Some of the most stubborn allergies show up on the hands. Soaps, cleansers, detergents, gloves, plastics, and hundreds of metals, plants and chemicals could be the reason for the rash.

The following pages include a discussion of three common forms of contact dermatitis: poison ivy dermatitis, cosmetic contact dermatitis, and occupational dermatoses.

POISON IVY DERMATITIS

"Leaflets three, let it be" is an old poetic warning. To which let me add my own unpoetic, "Don't be rash with poison ivy."

The three-leafer is the most common cause of contact dermatitis in the United States. The typical poison ivy plant grows in most of the central and eastern parts of the country as low-lying shrubs or high-climbing aerial plants. (It sometime grows as ornamental shrubs in gardens!) The poison ivy plant has thin, pale stems upon which are three leaflets. If you suspect that a plant is poison ivy, grasp it with a piece of folded white paper and crush it. If it's poison ivy, the sap on the paper will turn black in five minutes.

Other related plants that can cause "poison" rashes are poison oak and poison sumac. Poison oak grows mainly in the West, and poison sumac flourishes along the eastern seaboard. The plants grow as vines on walls, fences, trees, telephone poles, and other vines, or as ground shrubs of various sizes.

Despite its name, poison ivy is not a poison. And, contrary to popular myth, it is not contagious. The sap of these "poison" plants all contain an allergic substance, one that can cause skin rashes in susceptible individuals. You get the rash by rubbing against or in some other manner exposing yourself to the plant. The allergic chemical in the plant, an oil called *urushiol*, acts as a foreign material (antigen) on the skin, stirring up a defensive mechanism in your body. Your skin responds by forming certain "protective" cells (antibodies). This combination of the foreign and protective substances stimulates your immune system resulting in the redness, blisters, and itching that we call poison ivy dermatitis.

You don't have to come in direct contact with a poison ivy plant to develop a poison ivy rash. You cat get it by touching shoes, various articles of clothing, sports equipment, and other objects that came in contact with poison ivy. You can get it by petting an animal whose fur may have been contaminated from bushes. And you can get poison ivy dermatitis on your eyelids and face just by burning the leaves, due to active material in the smoke.

Following contact with the plant, a rash will develop in almost everyone. If you have a history of previous poison ivy episodes, then your rash will appear within a few hours after exposure. If you have never had poison ivy dermatitis before, the rash may take two to three weeks to develop after the initial exposure.

The rash that develops from poison ivy begins as redness, followed by small blisters, usually in streaks, accompanied by itching. The exposed areas of the skin are most often affected— the hands, forearms, and face. The eruption may become severe, with marked swelling of the eyelids, widespread skin involvement, fever, and secondary infection.

Although poison ivy dermatitis is not contagious, the chemical responsible for the rash remains active after the initial contact. You yourself can spread the rash to other parts of your body within the first hour after contact. After one hour on the skin, however, this chemical changes so that no further contamination will occur. Inanimate objects, such as clothing and camping equipment, can retain the substance for months, thus producing the rash when least expected.

Poison ivy dermatitis knows no season. More cases, however, occur in late spring and early summer, when the plant sap is most abundant in the stem and leaves.

Treatment for poison ivy dermatitis depends upon the severity of the eruption.

If you know you have come in contact with one of these "poison" plants, thoroughly wash yourself with soap and water as soon after exposure as possible. Preferably within ten minutes. While this will not prevent an outbreak of the rash, it may help minimize the spread. Make sure you wash under your fingernails, too. And wash all contaminated clothing, sports equipment, and animals.

In mild, fairly localized cases, warm water compresses and plain calamine lotion (do not use other, over-the-counter "poison ivy remedies") will help dry up the tiny blisters and relieve the itching.

In more severe and extensive cases, it is advisable to see a dermatologist. The latest approved treatment, and one which promises to stop the rash in its tracks, is high-dose therapy with cortisone-like drugs. This should be done early, as soon as the little bumps appear on the skin, and before the allergenic substance has a chance to sensitize the skin cells.

The treatment for mild cases of poison ivy dermatitis is the same as the treatment for allergy rashes. See page 94.

To protect against poison ivy dermatitis, wear protective clothing when hiking or weeding: long sleeves, high socks, and gloves; and then carefully remove the protective clothing and wash them in soap and water.

ALLERGY RASHES DUE TO COSMETICS

In our society many women, and men, too, go to great lengths to look good and smell good. This pursuit is reinforced by the myriad products on the market that claim to help us retain our youthful, healthy looks.

If you are a young woman, how many products might you put on your face, hair, body, and nails before you leave the house? From the top:

On your hair you might use conditioner, color or tint, shampoo, creme rinse, setting lotion, mousse, and hair spray. Dye? Bleach? Relaxer? Permanent-wave solution? In the bath you might use soap, bath oil, bath oil beads, bath salts, powder, and body lotion. And on your face, for starters, soap or cleansing cream and astringent, perhaps followed by moisturizer, foundation base, tinted base, shading cream, highlighting cream, contour cream, toner, freshener, clarifier, blusher, blotter, face powder, and mineral water spray. Your eyes are next—eye shadow, eye liner, eyebrow pencil, eyebrow powder, and mascara. Eye circle concealer? False eyelashes and glue? Lash extenders? For your lips—gloss, rouge, and lip liner.

Your fingernails and toenails will require a cuticle cream, base coat, nail conditioner, nail hardener, nail lacquer, nail gloss, and quick-dry solution. Artificial nails, perhaps? And don't forget the depilatory, deodorant and antiperspirant, hand cream, feminine hygiene spray, and perfume.

Did I forget anything?

Would you believe that each product just mentioned, sixty in all, can cause a skin allergy, hair breakage, or nail discoloration? There are about 8,000 chemicals that go into the making of cosmetics. You may use a cosmetic product for years without developing a reaction and suddenly become allergic to any of a number of the chemicals and preservatives, lanolin, dyes, and fragrances in it. In fact there isn't a product on the market, including the so-called hypoallergenic varieties, that cannot at some time, on some person, produce an allergic reaction on the skin.

A rash—dermatitis—does not always occur over the area where you apply a cosmetic. Dermatitis of the eyelids or neck, for example, is often due to nail polish or hair spray.

Cosmetic dermatitis is common in young men, as well. The chief causes are shave creams, hair dye, hair tonics, adhesives for hair pieces, bronzers, moisturizers, deodorants, soaps, sunscreens, and clear nail polish.

How can you tell if you have an allergy to a cosmetic, and what can you do about it? Determine what new products you may have been exposed to just before your rash appeared, and then eliminate all possible irritants. Change soaps to a mild, white, perfume-free variety. (*Cetaphil Lotion* or *Lowila Cake* are excellent soap substitutes.) Stop all scented lotions, creams, and sprays. Don't use any cosmetics for a week, then gradually use them one at a time. Or, better yet, try to live without a lot of them. The fewer the chemicals you expose your skin to, the less chance of it being irritated or sensitized.

You should also consider culprits other than what you yourself might be using. Have you been around anyone who wore a new perfume, cologne, or other scented toiletries? Anything new at the beauty shop or barber? At work? At school? The possibilities are infinite.

If you are unable to pinpoint the cause of your rash, your dermatologist will have the proper knowledge and equipment to determine the cause. And unless you eliminate the cause, this allergy rash will forever plague you whenever you are exposed to your Nemesis.

OCCUPATIONAL DERMATOSES

At last count, there were almost 10 million people working in almost 60,000 forms of employment, a staggering number of occupations. And there are literally thousands of different chemical, physical and biological agents in these 60,000 occupations that can be responsible for contact dermatitis and other skin ailments.

The skin has many functions, not the least of which is to protect us from a hostile environment that includes germs, irritants, blows, chemicals, temperature changes, and radiation. Yet despite the ability of the skin to withstand many of these onslaughts, it is still the most commonly injured organ.

Here are a few facts:

- Skin eruptions account for about 75 percent of all medical diseases compensated for and are the number one in-plant cause of lost time in industry.
- Fully ten percent of all skin diseases in the general population are industrial in origin.
- The cost of skin diseases due to occupational exposure runs into the hundreds of millions of dollars a year in medical expenses and lost time on the job.
- Four out of five cases of occupational contact dermatitis involve only the hands.
- Those who have suffered from eczema in childhood tend to be more prone to occupational contact dermatitis than others. Their hands frequently become aggravated in occupations such as hairdressing and machine operating.

Occupational dermatitis is defined as a "contact dermatitis for which exposure at work can be shown to be the main cause or one of the factors contributing to its occurrence." Direct causes of occupational or industrial skin diseases can be divided into seven groups:

1. Chemicals, the most frequent cause, include strong acids and alkalis, solvents, cutting oils, gases, and salts. All of these can injure the skin on direct contact, producing various kinds of rashes, while other chemicals, such as

those found in leather, lacquer or rubber, can cause rashes that are allergic in nature.

2. Mechanical factors, caused by pressure or friction (prolonged use of pneumatic tools, such as air hammers and chisels) are responsible for cuts, bruises, calluses, and the like. Fiberglas can produce a mechanical irritation and an itchy rash.

3. Physical agents in the form of excessive heat, sunlight, wind, and cold can cause burns, sunburn, allergic reactions, and frostbite.

4. Bacterial and fungal infections can occur among meat handlers, farmers, and grocers.

5. Insect bites and stings among outside workers are common dermatologic afflictions.

6. Bites from snakes and wild animals may arise in zookeepers, outdoor workers, garbage men, and mailpersons.

7. Poisonous plants and woods, as well as other vegetation, can cause skin problems among gardeners, farmers, road builders, surveyors, and telephone workers.

There are hundreds of products and chemicals in industry that can cause dermatitis in otherwise healthy people. Almost anything can be responsible, but certain occupations are more susceptible than others to contact dermatitis.

The following are some common occupations and material used in these jobs that are responsible for rashes:

Artists: Turpentine, solvents, clay, plaster, paint, sprays, ink.
Auto mechanics: Solvents, cutting oils, paints, cleansers, greases, kerosene, lacquer.
Bakers: Flour, spices, cinnamon, nuts, lemon, flavorings.
Barbers and hairdressers: Soaps, shampoos, permanent-wave solutions, hair dyes, rubber gloves, bleaching agents.
Bartenders: Detergents, cleansers, citrus fruits.
Bookbinders: Glue, plastics, solvents.
Building tradespeople: Cement, epoxy resins, rubber and leather gloves.
Butchers: Detergents, meats.
Canning industry: Juices, dyes, preservatives, brine.
Carpenters: Polishes, glue, solvents, cleansers, adhesives, wood.

Clerks and office workers: Carbon paper, glue, typewriter ribbons, copy paper, rubber, nickel.

Cooks: Meat and vegetable juices, spices, detergents.

Dentists and dental technicians: Resins, acrylics, fluxes, mercury, rubber gloves, local anesthetics.

Dry cleaners: Benzene, turpentine, carbon tetrachloride.

Electricians: Rubber, tape, glues, solvents, soldering flux.

Exterminators: Arsenic, DDT, formaldehyde, pyrethrum.

Florists and gardeners: Fertilizer, pesticides, plants (tulips, chrysanthemums, narcissus).

Food industry: Vegetables, spices, rubber gloves, detergents.

Foundry work: Oils, hand cleansers, resins, plastics.

Garment and millinery industries: Dyes, turpentine, benzene.

Groceries and delicatessen: Dyes on labels, insecticides, cardboard boxes, paper bags.

Hospital workers: Soaps, detergents, disinfectants, rubber gloves, penicillin, streptomycin.

Household workers: Detergents, polishes, solvents, rubber gloves, sprays.

Jewelers: Solvents, nickel, enamel, chrome.

Laundry workers: Detergents, bleaches, solvents, turpentine, starch, antiseptics, soap.

Manicurists: Nail polish, acrylic nails, cosmetics.

Masons: Cement, acids, resins, rubber and leather gloves.

Medical technicians and nurses: Detergents, plastics, solvents, antibiotics, antiseptics, anesthetics, formalin, rubber gloves.

Metal workers: Cutting oils, cleansers, solvents.

Painters: Turpentine, thinners, solvents, paints, dyes and adhesives in wallpaper.

Paper manufacturers: Glues and pastes.

Photographers: Acids, solvents, formaldehyde, dyes, color developers.

Plastic industry: Solvents, acids, additives, hardeners.

Platers: Solvents, paints, chromium, acids and alkalis.

Plumbers: Oils, hand cleansers, rubber, cement, nickel.

Printers: Solvents, glues, turpentine, paper finishes.

Rubber workers: Solvents, rubber, dyes, tars.

Shoemakers: Solvents, glues, leather, rubber, turpentine, cement, polishes.

Sporting goods: Lead, rubber, nickel, chrome, leather, dyes.

Textile workers: Solvents, bleaching agents, fibers, dyes, finishes.

Theatrical profession: Cosmetics, dyes, glues.
Undertakers: Formaldehyde, embalming fluids.
Welders: Oil, chromium, nickel.
Window shade makers: Paint, benzene, shellac.
Woodworkers: Woods, turpentine, lacquers, varnish, tars, paints.

What is particularly sobering is that we can control and prevent fully *90 percent* of all occupational dermatoses by using protective clothing and cleansers.

The cure of contact dermatitis depends largely on detection and removal of the cause. This search for the causes can be one of the most intricate tasks confronting an allergist or dermatologist. But once we have discovered the causative agent, it is relatively easy to cure the rash and prevent recurrences.

TREATING ALLERGY RASHES

For a severe, oozing allergy rash over one specific area (for example, poison ivy or nail polish dermatitis), use warm cloths soaked with the following:

Bluboro Powder (Herbert)

Follow the Directions on the package and use as compresses as described on page 217.

For a rash that has spread all over the body, take soothing baths in either:

Alpha Keri Bath Oil (Westwood)
Nutraderm Bath Oil (Owen)

Directions are on the bottles.

When the oozing areas have begun to dry up, stop the compresses and baths and try one of the following creams or lotions to give you some relief from the itching and to help soften and smooth the skin:

Hytone Cream 0.5 (Dermik)
Sarna Lotion (Stiefel)
Schamberg's Lotion (C&M Pharmacal)

Directions: Apply every three to four hours and after the bath.

Never use soap on any allergy rash. Instead, use the following cleanser or soap substitute for getting clean:

Cetaphil Lotion (Owen/Galderma)
Lowila Cake (Westwood)

Allergy rashes almost always itch. Take either of the following antihistamines every four hours as necessary to control the itching:

Chlor-Trimeton Tablets [4 mg] (Schering)

Dimetane [4 mg] Robins

Be sure to follow the directions for use and read the cautions on the label.

HAIR AND HAIR CARE

Hair—our crowning glory.

And yet, depending on where it grows, how much, and upon whom, hair can be either a blessing or curse.

We cut it, shave it, twirl it, comb it, and brush it to make it appear longer and more abundant. Some of us tease, tint, dye, bleach, spray, iron, and frost it. We straighten curly hair, and we curl straight hair. Blonds become brunettes, and vice versa.

We tear our hair. We split hairs. We let our hair down. We make our hair stand on end, and we get into someone else's hair.

What is this culturally, socially, and sexually significant ornamental appendage we refer to as hair? It is a nonliving, protein fiber, a strong, elastic thread, arising from a long indentation, a follicle, or "pore," in the skin.

Hair is dead. Although it is as integral a component of the body as our skin, once it has emerged from the follicle, it is no longer nourished by a blood supply or by any other life-giving bodily fluids.

What, then, is its purpose? Thousands of years ago our forebears were covered with hair in much the same manner as the monkeys and apes. It was a protective barrier against the elements: the sun, the wind, extremes of heat and cold, rain and snow, insects. It also acted as a type of cushion to protect against the force of bumps, abrasions, and blows in battle.

Gradually, as we evolved, our need for hair diminished. We developed clothing to protect us from the ravages of nature and soon lost most of our redundant body hair. Today, except for our eyebrows and eyelashes which act as a sieve against insects, dust, and other irritants, hair serves no biological function.

Hair varies in color, texture, length, and type among different races. It is second only to skin as a physical sign of racial difference. Asians, Eskimos, and native Americans have sparse facial and body hair and straight, coarse, dark hairs on their heads. African blacks have slightly more body hair and woolly or wiry hair on their scalps. American blacks, who are often mixtures of other races, have straight, wavy, curly, fine, or coarse hair on their heads. Whites have more body hair than any other race and have curly, wavy, or straight, fine hair on their heads.

As a rule, we each have three types of hair: the long, soft, terminal hairs, such as those on the scalp, armpits, and pubic region; the short, stiff, coarse hairs of the eyelids, eyebrows, nose, and ears; and the soft, fine, downy fuzz (known as lanugo or vellus hairs) which covers much of the rest of our bodies. Our only "hairless" regions are the palms and soles, the lips, the nipples, and certain parts of the genitals.

All of us are born with a fixed number of hair follicles which remain with us on our heads, in our armpits, on our faces and bodies, for an entire lifetime. Each hair follicle is supplied by one or more oil glands which produce a secretion that gives your hair its richness and gloss. The number of hair follicles, and, therefore, hairs, is inherited. In other words, if your parents had 100,000 hairs on their heads, the chances are that you will have approximately the same number.

Blonds may or may not have more fun than everyone else, but they do have more hair. They average about 120,000 scalp hairs, while brunettes have about 100,000, and redheads only 80,000. To compensate for this disparity, however, blond hairs are thin (fine) and red hairs are thick (coarse). If we weighed the total number of scalp hairs from an average blond, they would weigh roughly the same as those of a redhead! Although fine hair is a nuisance and a bother, blonds, since they have more hair on their heads, can afford to lose more; and, because there's more of it, fine hair has a tendency to go gray more slowly.

Hair loss on the scalp in normal, healthy people varies from about 50 to 120 strands daily. In other words, in the course of a year you'll lose about 30,000 hairs from your scalp. All of these hairs are constantly being replaced, at least until the aging process and certain hormonal changes begin to occur.

Most scalp hairs grow about one-half inch a month, so it takes only about two years to grow shoulder-length hair. Each strand of hair, however, does not grow indefinitely. If you never had your hair cut, your hair would only grow about two-and-one-half feet. After a period of time (usually two to four years), the hair follicle that produces the individual hair gets tired and stops working. The strand stops growing and eventually falls out, to be replaced by a new "working" hair when the follicle has revived and renewed itself.

Hair grows faster in warm weather, slows down during illness or pregnancy, and falls out more in autumn when "the leaves on the trees begin to drop." Contrary to popular myths and superstitions, hair does not grow thicker or faster when cut or shaved. Nor does it grow after death.

The following sections cover some basics that can help you have healthier looking hair as well as cope with some common conditions that affect our scalp and hair, such as dandruff, seborrheic dermatitis, too little hair, and too much hair.

HAIR CARE

Compare your hair to a cashmere sweater. How long would that sweater last if you constantly were to wash, shampoo, comb, brush, color, tint, bleach, tease, straighten, curl, roll, pull, twist, and twirl it? What if you constantly exposed it to the sun, wind, rain, snow, and sleet and to extremes of heat and cold? How about if you wore it swimming in polluted lakes and streams and chlorinated pools? And then you got it steamed, ironed, sprayed, flipped, oiled, wound, feathered, swirled, dipped, stripped, frosted, perfumed, frizzed, fuzzed, matted, braided, and waxed, and then blown dry by 1500 watts of hot air? How long would it last? A month? A week?

Your hair goes through this and more. Yet, barring certain diseases and conditions, it lasts a lifetime.

Taking good care of your hair, however, can make a big difference in how it looks during its "lifetime." Healthy-looking, attractive hair requires consistently good care and conditioning, good diet, and good exercise. It requires keeping stress and emotional tensions to a minimum. (Remember, I did not say *healthy* hair; I said *healthy-looking* hair. How can something that's dead be healthy?)

Many young women (and, increasingly, men) consult a dermatologist because they're concerned about a change in the growth or appearance of their hair. More often than not, the change is the result of abuse, rather than disease, causing the hair to break off easily.

What causes breakage of hair? Often, it is related to physical damage. Here are some factors that can physically "injure" your hair:

- Using brushes with sharp bristles
- Using metal or plastic combs
- Braiding your hair tightly
- Winding your hair too tightly
- Using brush rollers
- Back-combing
- Repeatedly wetting and blow-drying your hair
- Other forms of repeated manipulation of your hair
- Wearing tight hats, caps, and headbands

Chemical injury is probably the most common cause of hair breakage. When the outer keratin layer of the hair shaft (the cuticle) is repeatedly exposed to chemical attack from bleaches, hair straighteners, permanent hair dyes, thioglycolate wave solutions, etc., the hair develops a stiff, strawlike feel, making it more susceptible to breakage.

To prevent hair breakage and maintain a healthier-looking head of hair, avoid excessive manipulation and physical injury to the hair shaft as much as possible. Hair normally "wears out," and increased manipulation, in whatever form, speeds up the process. Here are some specific tips:

- Brush and comb less often. (The so-called 100-strokes-a-day brushing or combing is *not* good for your hair.)
- Don't back-comb
- No braids or pony-tails
- Use pure bristle brushes and hard rubber (Ace) combs
- Don't wear tight hats, caps, or headbands
- Use a mild, gentle shampoo

- Use creme rinses
- Trim split and damaged ends

A word about shampooing:

Good hair care begins with shampooing. The frequency of shampooing is an individual affair. You may shampoo daily or oftener, if need be, without harming the hair or hair follicle in any way.

If your hair is oily, or if you live in the city where you are constantly exposed to inordinate amounts of dust, grease, grime, soot, and other chemical pollutants, you should shampoo often. And with a good commercial shampoo, not with bar soap.

An important and little stressed fact about shampooing is that to derive any benefit from it, the shampoo should be massaged into the entire scalp for *at least* five minutes, preferably longer, using fairly hot water. Thorough rinsing is a must. For those who like a creme rinse, I recommend using it in moderation, only small amounts to prevent the "greasies."

If you blow dry your hair, follow the manufacturer's directions and make sure to keep the blow dryer at least six inches away from your hair.

HAIR CARE PRODUCTS

There are dozens of shampoos flooding the shelves of your drugstore and supermarket. There are shampoos for normal hair, dry hair, and oily hair. For dandruff, psoriasis, eczema. For "thinning" hair. For hair repair. For infants and children. And there are shampoos containing sulfur, salicylic acid, tar, zinc, and selenium. Any or all of them may be good for you. It's basically a matter of choosing one that works.

For normal scalp and hair, try:

Neutrogena Shampoo (Neutrogena)

Purpose Brand Shampoo (Johnson & Johnson)

For oily scalp and hair, try:

Pernox Shampoo (Westwood)

Ionil Shampoo (Owen)

DHS Shampoo (Person & Covey)

For creme rinses, try either of the following:

Ionil Cream Rinse (Owen)

DHS Conditioning Rinse (Person & Covey)

DANDRUFF

"Nothing stops dandruff like a blue serge suit." Blue serge may be a little before your time, but the saying still has more than a speck of truth to it.

Dandruff is a normal condition. Everyone has it to some degree. It's only when the scaling or flaking of dandruff shows up like stardust on the collar of that dark suit or dress that you may become embarrassed and concerned.

To understand dandruff, you have to know a little about the epidermis, the upper layer of the skin. Like all cells in the body, skin cells are manufactured constantly to replace those that have outlived their usefulness and died. In normal skin, the process for a cell to be born, move to the outer edge of the skin surface, and then flake off takes about a month. Dead cells are being continually sloughed off as new ones are being pushed up from the deeper layers in a never ending process of cell division. This cycle gives rise to the tiny, scaly flakes you continuously shed from the entire skin surface.

On the scalp, you can control this normal, periodic scaling by frequent shampooing with everyday commercial shampoos. In the abnormal process, however, the cells are born and die at a much faster rate, giving rise to lots of flaking and sometimes even redness and itching. To control this moderately severe type of dandruff will probably require other than the usual over-the-counter antidandruff remedies.

No one really knows what causes this flaking to get out of control. Many theories have been proposed: hormone imbalance, germs (bacteria and fungi) living on the scalp, excessive production of oil from the oil glands, dietary indiscretions and deficiencies, allergies, poor hygiene, irritation and inflammation as a result of various cosmetics and chemicals applied to the scalp, hereditary influences, and emotional stress. One rarely sees dandruff in children under the age of twelve, which leads us to suspect that some type of hormone influences the condition. There is no clear-cut proof, however, to support any of these theories.

We do know, however, that dandruff is not contagious (you can't pick it up from someone's comb), it does not lead to any serious scalp problem, and it does NOT cause baldness.

There are dozens of shampoos that are commercially available for the relief of simple dandruff. But remember, you never really get "rid" of dandruff, since your scalp makes a new supply of flakes about every three days.

No one shampoo is good for everybody. Where you live, the type of water in your home, as well as your particular kind of hair, all play a role in the effectiveness of a particular shampoo.

Medicated shampoos usually contain either sulfur, zinc, selenium, tar, or a combination of these. Your pharmacist can offer you a variety of these preparations. Find the one you like, the one you feel is most effective, and stick with it.

If your dandruff is persistent and doesn't respond to frequent and conscientious shampooing, check with your dermatologist. You may have seborrheic dermatitis or psoriasis or some other condition that requires medical expertise.

TREATING DANDRUFF

To take care of an occasional few flakes of dandruff, try any of the following shampoos:

Sebulex Conditioning Shampoo (Westwood)

Selsun Blue (Abbott)

DHS Zinc Shampoo (Herbert)

For stubborn scaling and itching of the scalp, one of the following tar shampoos might help:

Ionil-T Plus Shampoo (Owen)

Sebutone Shampoo (Westwood)

Polytar Shampoo (Stiefel)

Following your tar shampoo, try the following conditioner:

T/Gel Conditioner (Neutrogena)

The following are two medicated hair dressings for dandruff and related scaly conditions of the scalp:

Sebucare (Westwood)

Drest Gel (Dermik)

Directions for use are on each tube.

SEBORRHEIC
DERMATITIS

Seborrheic dermatitis is a fancy name for what I refer to as "dandruff of the skin."

Characterized by symmetrically distributed, red, scaly, and greasy patches, seborrheic dermatitis is a condition, not really a disease, that a dermatologist can diagnosis just by looking at you. It doesn't take fancy blood tests, sophisticated laboratory analyses, or microscopic examination of a piece of skin to prove conclusively that you do, indeed, have seborrheic dermatitis. All it takes is a dermatologist's scrupulous eye.

Like hundreds of other skin ailments, no one knows what causes seborrheic dermatitis. And, as with so many other disorders, there are many theories concerning the "why" of this common, but troublesome problem. These theories include the following:

- a hormonal imbalance
- a hereditary predisposition
- dietary indiscretions and obesity
- drugs (Thorazine, Haldol, Navane)
- environmental factors
- germs
- emotional stress and tension, worry, loss of sleep
- certain nervous disorders.

A recent theory proposes that seborrheic dermatitis results from a defect in your body's defense against certain germs that live on the surface of your skin. Actually, no one knows.

There is a condition in infants called "cradle cap," where the scalp is covered with thick, yellowish-brown, greasy crusts, and where the hair becomes sticky and matted. This common disorder is thought to be due to leftover hormones that have been passed on to the susceptible infant from his or her mother. These maternal hormones act to stimulate the sebaceous (oil) glands in the scalp, with the result that there is a marked production of an oily secretion, sebum. This sebum is responsible for "cradle cap," the earliest manifestation of seborrheic dermatitis.

Shortly after birth, activity in these sebaceous glands diminishes, with the result that you will almost never have seborrheic dermatitis during your childhood. When you reach puberty, however, your developing sex glands begin to stimulate these quiescent "oil formers," which then increase in size and become very active. If you have seborrheic dermatitis, you will notice that the condition begins on your scalp in the form of redness and diffuse scaling.

In addition to this "heavy dandruff," you'll find that your hair gets greasy and your scalp may itch. Scaly, pink, crust-like patches may begin to form around your hairline. Other areas of your body rich in oil glands often develop patches as well—your eyebrows, the areas over and behind your ears, your ear canals, the sides of your nose, and your forehead.

If you are a young man, you may develop these patches in your beard, your sideburns, and your mustache area. In certain cases, you may have the rash on your chest, back, and pubic region. Some people develop it in the body folds: the groins, the armpits, under the breasts, and in the bellybutton.

Your rash may or may not itch.

A special case of seborrheic dermatitis occurs when the margins of the eyelids become red and covered with small white scales or yellowish crusts.

Since seborrheic dermatitis is a chronic and recurring condition, flare-ups at odd moments are common. These occur more often in colder months.

Treatment of seborrheic dermatitis is directed at minimizing the symptoms, rather than curing the disorder permanently. Persistent, regular, and repeated treatment should give you good control over this annoying ailment.

Here are a dozen suggestions for managing and living with your seborrheic dermatitis:

1. Shampoo frequently—daily if at all possible. Frequent shampooing is the first rule in treating seborrheic dermatitis. (Specific shampoos are mentioned at the end of this chapter.)
2. Since the patches of seborrheic dermatitis are prone to secondary infection by bacteria and other germs, keep your skin clean by washing carefully and regularly using a mild, gentle soap like *Lowila Cake* or a cleanser such as *Cetaphil Lotion.*
3. Keep "cool." Avoid stress and emotional tension.
4. Get plenty of rest.
5. Eat a well-balanced diet.
6. Avoid greasy foods and alcoholic beverages.
7. If you are overweight, try to lose those extra pounds.
8. Avoid greasy cosmetics and oily moisturizers.
9. If it itches, try not to scratch.
10. Small amounts of sunlight usually help, but since the sun's rays have potential serious side effects, expose yourself carefully and in moderation.

11. If you are under the care of a dermatologist, follow his or her instructions for the proper use of topical medications.
12. Avoid those over-the-counter remedies that have not been recommended by your doctor.

Specific treatment for seborrheic dermatitis will depend on the location of the rash and how extensive it is. In mild cases of seborrheic dermatitis, when the scalp is the only area that is affected, frequent and conscientious shampooing with an antidandruff shampoo may be all that is necessary. In the more stubborn cases, and when the patches are extensive, you should consult your dermatologist.

The time-honored topical medications used in treating seborrheic dermatitis are sulfur, tar, salicylic acid, and cortisone-type creams and lotions. Many of these are prescription items that must be prescribed by your dermatologist.

A few of the over-the-counter remedies he or she may suggest for the milder cases of seborrheic dermatitis are various shampoos and topical creams and lotions such as those mentioned below.

For the stubborn variety of this common ailment, other methods, injections, stronger cortisone-like creams and lotions, and other topical preparations, may be necessary.

TREATING SEBORRHEIC DERMATITIS

When treating seborrheic dermatitis, it's important to shampoo as often as possible, preferably daily. Try any of the following shampoos:

Ionil-T Plus Shampoo (Owen)
Sebutone Shampoo (Westwood)
Polytar Shampoo (Stiefel)
Directions for use are on each label.

Apply a hydrocortisone preparation to the affected areas 2 or 3 times daily. Use either of the following:

Hytone Cream 0.5% (Dermik)
Cort-Aid Ointment (Upjohn)
Directions for use are on each container.

Use a mild soap substitute or cleanser for your face, such as:

Lowila Cake (Westwood)
Cetaphil Lotion (Owen/Galderma)

MALE BALDNESS

"Ugly are hornless bulls, a field without grass is an eyesore,
So is a tree without leaves, so is a head without hair."

                                   Ovid, *The Art of Love.*

Male baldness may be a joke on TV, in the movies, and at parties, but for the many young men who face the prospect of premature baldness, and who literally grasp at every lost hair, it is no joke at all. It can be a source of great anxiety, a personal loss, and a profoundly depressing experience, forcing a young man to revise his self-image. To some the fountain of youth is no more than a head full of dead protein threads.

Would it comfort you to know that Caesar was bald? Do Telly Savalas and Curly look as if they're suffering? Mr. Clean?

The hirsute male has forever been a symbol of virility and physical strength. The biblical Samson, the Greek Hercules, Zeus, and Poseidon were men and gods of prodigious strength and were usually represented as powerful, hairy, and bearded. But so are gorillas!

Male pattern baldness, which continues to be one of man's greatest fears, affects well over half the adult male population in the United States and is so common that we consider some degree of hair loss in adult males as normal.

Would it console you to know that hair loss has absolutely no adverse effect on virility? Or on potency? Or on strength? Would it help you to know there are some disadvantages to long hair? It can obstruct your vision. It collects dandruff and, occasionally, small creatures such as lice! The only harmful effect of premature hairloss is psychological. It may encourage loss of confidence and, with it, anxiety, stress, and depression.

The cause and extent of male baldness, while not completely understood, depend on three factors: inheritance, age, and male hormones. If your parents and/or grandparents had this bald trait, the chances are that you will inherit it. Once begun, it is a progressive condition; the older you get, the more hair you will lose.

You'll be surprised to know that when you get bald, you actually don't lose any of your hair. In fact, you go to the grave with the same number of hair follicles with which you were born! What the balding man loses are the longer, darker, coarser hairs which have been replaced with soft, downy fuzz, called vellus hairs.

Medical science so far has been helpless in reversing, arresting, or curing this pattern. There is, however, a great deal of research going on in an attempt to fatten up and lengthen those downy, vellus hairs.

And, lest you be sadly misled, there are no salves, lotions, shampoos, vitamins, or natural food supplements that will grow hair where there are no hair follicles. Hair "restorers" are for the birds, not for the scalp.

Years ago, it was demonstrated that the female hormone estrogen, when rubbed into the scalp, could lengthen the peach fuzz appreciably and slow down or reduce the rate of pattern baldness. Men, however, should think twice about the side effects of estrogen. Do you want larger breasts? A high-pitched voice? A diminished sexual appetite? Or would you rather grin and bare it?

There is, however, a new drug, minoxidil, that has shown some promise. Currently, it is being used orally for people who are afflicted with severe high blood pressure. How minoxidil helps high blood pressure, or how it helps grow hair, is not precisely known. It probably acts as a vasodilator, a chemical that expands blood vessels, bringing nourishing blood to normally-deprived hair follicle cells.

Among minoxidil's many undesirable side effects is hypertrichosis, the growth of excess hair, which is noted in about 80 percent of the patients taking the drug. What dermatologists have done has been to "tame" this powerful chemical and have fashioned it into a lotion which, when rubbed into bald spots, grows hair in those areas.

While there have been some dramatic results (and claims) using minoxidil topically, the results and potential harmful side effects have not yet been fully evaluated. The latest reports show that young men, under the age of 26, who are using this product, do much better than older men. It rarely works at all for a receding hairline. It can best restore hair on the crown of the head but not at the temples. The hairs, if any, that do grow, are little more than wispy. No one in the studies that were performed developed a full head of hair. The product, Rogaine, is expensive and must be used forever—when it is discontinued, any hair that had begun to grow will fall out within three or four months. Adverse side effects including fainting, vomiting, rapid heart beat, and difficulty in breathing.

So what does that leave for the despondent young man? A hair transplant? A wig? Or the confidence in knowing that bald may be beautiful. That the highbrow and the egghead, the marks of internal wisdom, are "in."

FEMALE HAIR LOSS

Are young American women becoming bald?

There is no clear-cut answer to this pressing problem. We do know, however, that in the past few decades there have been more and more complaints in dermatologists' offices from young women about hair loss, steady, progressive, diffuse, mysterious hair loss. There are very few medical conditions that produce more emotional trauma than thinning of scalp hair in young and middle-aged, healthy women.

Years ago, doctors rarely saw cases of female baldness. But recently, young women have begun to notice a gradual and progressive increase in the number of hairs lost with each brushing and combing—more hair on the comb, more hair in the brush, more hair in the wash basin. And, after months or years, a realization that there has occurred visible thinning, a euphemism for baldness.

The healthy scalp loses between 50 and 120 hairs daily. This loss, let me reassure you, is balanced out by continuous regrowth. When the rate of hair loss, however, exceeds the rate of new growth, thinning and balding become apparent.

As a rule, there really is not an excessive amount of hair loss, rather there is an underproduction of new hair. This lack of production of new, viable hair can be due to a dozen different reasons.

The major factors in what the dermatologist terms "female pattern baldness" are hormonal changes, heredity, and the aging process. Hormonal changes are those that occur after childbirth and with certain types of endocrine tumors and imbalances (thyroid trouble, ovarian problems, and other hormone conditions). In addition, if you are taking the low-dose birth control pill, you may be experiencing hair loss.

Hereditary factors also play a strong role in pattern baldness. If your mother or grandmother had sparse hair, it is likely that you (and possibly your daughter) may suffer from the same deficiency.

Finally, the aging process (due to diminished production of female hormones) is a strong factor in female hair loss. After producing for so many decades, the hair follicles become weak, tired, and sluggish. Some of them fade away and produce no more, one of the prices we must pay for growing old.

Other causes of thinning and balding in our modern women are due to environmental changes and the products used for beautification. Here are some examples:

- Mechanical tension and violence on the hair shaft due to new hair styles and cosmetic aids. These cause injury to the hair follicle and, when prolonged, interfere with the scalp's circulation. Examples include unusual stretching, pulling, and teasing, brush rollers and curlers, tight, restrictive hair styles, vigorous combing and brushing, hot combs, braiding, and ponytails. Sharp-toothed nylon and metal combs and brushes also cause mechanical injury to the hair shaft and follicle.
- Excessive chemical exposure associated with hair styling (for example, cold-wave solutions, bleaches, and hair straighteners), and increased exposure to synthetic detergents and other additives in commercial shampoos, dyes, and hair sprays.
- Pollutants in our water supply (pesticides and insecticides), in our air (radioactive fallout and other forms of radiation), in sprays and other inhalants, in our food (dyes, additives, and various drugs and hormones given to cattle and poultry), and increased exposure to chemicals of all sorts.
- Nutritional deficiencies, such as those seen in "crash dieters," in vegetarians who may develop protein malnutrition, and in those suffering from iron-deficiency anemia.
- General anesthesia during surgical operations.
- Various drugs used to treat cancer, and anticoagulants (blood thinners) used in heart disease.
- Excessive smoking (a more recent suspect).
- Emotional stress and tension, which are believed to impair the circulation of the hair follicle.

What's a woman to do? Here are a few basic do's and don't's for healthy hair:

- Shampoo your hair regularly, daily if at all possible.
- If you comb and brush your hair, use only pure bristle brushes and hard rubber (Ace) combs. Don't use the plastic or metal varieties.
- Reduce excessive mechanical manipulation of the hair shaft. Avoid teasing and ratting, vigorous combing and brushing, tight, restrictive hairstyles, tight braids and ponytails, and excessive hot-combing. Hair responds best to gentle care.
- Avoid excessive bleaching, dyeing, and hair straightening.
- Keep up your general health, avoid crash diets, and cut down on smoking.
- If you are taking the low-dose birth control pill, ask your gynecologist if you may change these to the higher-dose variety.
- Avoid emotional stress and tension.
- Don't be misled by those advertisements and commercials for potions and unguents that promise to grow hair. There ain't no such animal.
- Finally, if your situation does not improve, see your dermatologist. There may be some infection, some hormonal imbalance, or some medication that you have been taking that might be responsible.

And remember, women don't get bald the way men do. While you may have to get used to a thinner crop when you are in your forties, it is highly unlikely that you will lose all of your "crowning glory."

ALOPECIA AREATA

"Bogie noticed a bare spot on his cheek where his beard was not growing. The one spot increased to several—then he'd wake in the morning and find clumps of hair on the pillow. . . . A visit to the doctor was in order. The verdict was that he had a disease known as alopecia areata—in layman's terms, hair falls out. . . . His next film was going to be *The Treasure of the Sierra Madre* with John Huston, and he'd have to wear a wig . . ."

—From "Lauren Bacall By Myself"

It goes by the lilting name of alopecia areata, but patchy hair loss, as it's commonly called, would not be desirable by any name. Still, it can be treated, so don't despair.

Patchy hair loss is pretty much what it says it is, a condition of the scalp and other hairy areas of the body that begins with the sudden appearance of one or more small, round or oval bald patches which gradually enlarge over a period of weeks. It affects all age groups but is more common among children and young adults.

The bald patches appear rather quickly on an otherwise normal, healthy, hairy area. They do not itch, burn, or cause any pain. The scalp is the area most commonly affected, but alopecia areata can affect the beard, eyebrows, eyelashes, and any other hairy region as well. The hairs at the periphery of these balding patches are usually loose and easily pulled out.

In severe cases, patches on the scalp become so large that they merge to produce a total loss of all the scalp hair. This is alopecia totalis. In rare cases, the condition may progress until every hair of the entire body falls out—alopecia universalis. (Queen Elizabeth I of England contracted this condition in 1562 following her severe bout with smallpox. She was completely bald for the remainder of her life and resorted to wigs and other artifices.)

No one knows why the hair root on some people simply stops making hair. I explain to my patients that while the hair-growing "equipment" is in no way damaged, the "hair-growth switch" has been turned off. And once the switch has been turned back on, renewed hair growth will occur.

Theories have linked alopecia areata to certain hormonal changes, blows to the head, and severe emotional strain or shock. In some cases alopecia areata runs in families. The latest theory is that it may be an immune disorder, a type of "self allergy," where the body rejects its own tissue, in this case the hair follicle.

Fortunately, for many people, alopecia areata is a temporary, self-limiting disease. Even without treatment, the hairs often begin to grow back slowly after a few weeks or months. At first, the regrowth occurs as fine, downy white hairs. Eventually these hairs develop their normal texture and color. The course is erratic and unpredictable. As a rule, however, the greater the initial hair loss and the earlier in life it begins, the more likely it is to persist or recur.

Is there any treatment for alopecia areata? And can we turn the "switch" back on? Yes.

First of all, stop worrying. Make sure that your general health is good. Only your general physician can correct any deficiencies and give you a "clean bill of health."

Other treatments include injections of certain cortisone-like drugs directly into the bald patches. These injections are relatively painless and can hasten the regrowth and often prevent further hair loss. In severe cases, applying cortisone-type creams to the patches and covering them tightly with plastic or Saran Wrap may help.

A new topical drug, *Rogaine* (see page 107), also offers some promise in growing new hair in these balding patches, and your dermatologist can give you all the information regarding it.

Massage and hair tonics are worthless. If they do seem to help, it is only because time itself has allowed nature to do its job.

If you have an extensive and persistent case of alopecia areata, you may find that a hairpiece will give you peace of mind.

For further information regarding alopecia areata, write to:

National Alopecia Areata Foundation
714 C Street, Suite 202
San Rafael, California 94901
415/456-4644
Vicki Kalabokes, Executive Director

EXCESS HAIR

One of the unhappiest women I know is a young lady with an excess amount of dark hair on her upper lip, her chin, and her chest. She is not alone. There are thousands of young women with the same cosmetic problem—superfluous hair—hair that doesn't look sporty in the locker room, hair where nobody wants it.

Exactly what do we mean by excess hair? Not what most people believe.

Excess hair does *not* mean an increase in the number of hairs. Everyone is born with a fixed number of hairs on his or her body. This is genetically determined (inherited).

Hair grows on every portion of the skin except the palms and soles and a few other small areas. Most of these hairs are of the "peach-fuzz" variety (vellus hairs). Others are of the terminal variety—the long, thicker hairs of the scalp (Crystal Gayle, Rapunzel, David Lee Roth), the chest (mostly men), and the pubic region.

Excess hairiness results from the vellus hairs becoming longer, darker, and thicker in areas where one expects to have only peach-fuzz.

While excess hair may be due to many factors, for some groups of people it is the normal state of affairs. People from Southern Europe and Middle-Eastern cultures are much hairier than those from Northern Europe and Scandinavian countries; white people are hairier than black people; and Asians and American Indians are the least hairy of all.

Above and beyond this normal, constitutional hairy excess, there are those women who exhibit a far greater increase in the length and thickness of hair in certain areas which are usually reserved for the "peach-fuzz" variety: the upper lip, the chin, the sides of the face, the areas around the nipples, and the portion of the abdomen extending from the pubic region to the belly-button. (These are the areas normally associated with the male pattern hair growth.) This type of superfluous hair, or hypertrichosis, can be especially embarrassing to the young and otherwise confident woman, one of those "thousand natural shocks that flesh is heir to."

The causes of excess hair are many and varied. For those with a moderate degree of hairiness, the factors involved may be merely a part of normal growth and development.

The most common cause of excess hair growth in females is the aging process. Along about the time of menopause, women become deficient in the production of the female hormone estrogen. The decrease of this hormone gives rise to a relative increase in the male-type hormone (androgen), which is responsible for the slow, relentless proliferation of thick, dark hairs appearing on the upper lip, chin, and cheeks. And, at the same time, the beginning of the steady thinning of the scalp hair. These two processes seem to go hand in hand: more hair on the body, less on the scalp.

Stress and tension can also play a role in excess hair growth. The hair follicles are under the influence of various hormones and chemicals produced by the body. Emotional stress and tension often lead to a disturbance in the delicate balance of these hormones which, in turn, can result in a stimulation of the hair follicle leading to excess hair, not, however, on the head. These hormonal imbalances also can arise in connection with tumors and cysts of the ovaries, diseases of the adrenal glands, and abnormal functioning and tumors of other hormone-secreting glands, such as the thyroid or pituitary.

In addition, various drugs and medications can occasionally

produce hypertrichosis when taken over a period of time. These include drugs for epilepsy (Dilantin), cortisone-like drugs, and a host of others.

TREATMENT FOR EXCESS HAIR

Women who have excessive hair, on the body or the face, can suffer deep embarrassment. It isn't a problem you get rid of by saying "presto," but there are ways of dealing with the problem.

A normal woman (that is, one who has no hormonal disease or disturbance) can conceal or remove excess hair in a number of ways: bleaching, shaving, plucking with tweezers, depilatory creams and lotions, waxes, abrasive applicators, and electrolysis. All have their drawbacks and all, except electrolysis, are temporary measures.

Whether you will use any (or all) of the methods described below will depend upon the area (or areas) you intend to treat, your skin type, your tolerance to pain, your dexterity, your free time, and your pocketbook.

Bleaching: Bleaching with commercially-available products can conceal excessive, fine, fuzzy hair growth on the upper lip and forearms. It is most effective for small amounts of unwanted hair.

When done properly, bleaching is simple, safe, and painless. Repeated use of bleaching agents, however, can damage the hair shaft and cause temporary breakage. It can also irritate the skin. If you do use a bleach and develop a rash, try a different product.

Shaving: There is a popular myth that claims that if you shave or cut your hair, it will grow back faster, thicker, coarser, and darker. Don't believe it. There is no scientific evidence to support this old wives' tale. (If it were true, there would be very few bald men!)

The portion of hair emerging from the surface of the skin is nonliving, a dead protein thread. Cutting or shaving cannot influence the growing portion of your hair—the root—which occupies the hair follicle beneath the surface of the skin. Shaving is, however, a temporary measure and one must repeat it fairly often to avoid the stubbly feel and the "5 o'clock shadow" look.

If you shave with a safety razor, I recommend a clean, sharp, single-track blade. (Avoid using an old, ragged blade.) For a good shave, wet the hair thoroughly for at least two minutes with a lather shave cream which helps prevent evaporation. Do not shave too closely, as this practice can lead to ingrown hairs. And contrary to what you may have been taught, it is advisable to shave *with* the grain, *not* against it. This will also prevent ingrown hairs and subsequent infection.

If you use an electric shaver, try a preshave lotion which helps remove oil from the hair. You'll find that shaving is easier, and you'll be less likely to nick the skin.

Plucking (Tweezing): Plucking out hairs with tweezers is a popular and effective, although somewhat painful, way to remove temporarily scattered hairs on the face, chest, and eyebrows. Because of the discomfort and irritation, you should reserve this method for small areas of excess hair.

Plucking has no adverse side effects and, like other methods of temporary hair removal, will not cause the hairs to grow faster, coarser, or darker. Since the hair is removed at the root, it may grow back slower than hair that has been shaved off. Constant and repeated tweezing in the same area, however, can cause tiny, pitted scars.

When using the plucking method, make sure the skin and the tweezers are scrupulously clean to avoid infection. Also, *do not* pluck hairs from moles, warts, or other tumors. This can cause disagreeable and dangerous side effects: bleeding, infection, and change in the type of cell growth.

Hint: to minimize any pain, apply an ice cube to the area just before plucking.

Chemical Depilatories: Available in creams, liquids, and foams, these products weaken the chemical bonds of the hairs, causing them to break off or dissolve just below the surface of the skin. This is one of the best, easiest, and most popular methods for temporary removal of unwanted hair on the arms, legs, and underarm areas.

One word of caution: *do not* use these products on broken or abraded skin. It is also wise not to use them on very delicate areas, such as along the "bikini line" of the thighs or on the skin of the breasts.

The first time you use a chemical depilatory, try it on a "test" area first to make sure your skin isn't unusually sensitive to it. Then wash and thoroughly dry the area to be depilated. Apply the chemical and leave it on for a specific length of time, usually ten to fifteen minutes, depending on the directions given by the manufacturer. (If you leave it on longer than recommended, it can severely irritate your skin.) Then rinse the area thoroughly with clear, lukewarm water, using a washcloth if necessary, and pat dry. You can then apply a soothing, emollient cream or lotion because the chemical may dry out your skin.

The main advantage of chemical depilatories is that they are painless. They also break off hairs below the surface of the skin, so that regrowth is relatively slow and the hairs grow back soft, not stubbly.

Waxing: One of the oldest and least popular methods of temporary hair removal is molten wax. Hot, melted wax is poured onto the skin, left to cool and solidify, and then rapidly stripped off. The hairs which are embedded in the wax are plucked out as the wax is removed.

This type of hair removal is longer lasting than some of the other methods described. It takes about four to six weeks for waxed hair to grow back. However, there is always some degree of pain and skin irritation. Also, you cannot repeat this type of treatment until the hairs have grown out and are long enough to become embedded in the wax.

Abrasives: Pumice stones have been used for centuries to "wear off" excess hair. Although simple and inexpensive, this method of hair removal is rather tedious and uncomfortable and, therefore, not suitable for large areas.

Electrolysis: There is only one safe way to remove excess hair permanently: destroying the hair root with an electric current. This is called electrolysis.

Performed by a physician or trained electrologist, electrolysis consists of inserting a fine platinum or steel wire needle into the opening of the hair follicle. An electric current, transmitted down the needle, permanently destroys the hair root. The loosened hairs are then removed with tweezers. Once you destroy the root, the hair can no longer grow back.

While several types of electric current may be used, the basic procedure is the same. The results will depend upon the skill of the operator. Even in the most competent hands, however, electrolysis is a long, expensive, and tedious process. It is also somewhat painful, particularly on areas other than the face.

Electrolysis is most effective for the coarse, darker hairs, not the fine, "peach-fuzz," lanugo-type hairs. It has no effect on the cause of excessive hair growth; all it can do is destroy the existing hair.

Electrolysis is not one hundred percent effective, and repeated treatments are often necessary to destroy successfully all the unwanted hairs. There are several reasons for this. Some hair follicles are bent or crooked. The electrical current for the particular follicle may be insufficient (the higher the current, the greater the pain; therefore, the operator tries to "get away" with the smallest current that might do the job). Also, since the electrologist works below the surface of the skin, the insertion of the needle into the hair follicle is essentially a blind procedure and cannot be performed with absolute certainty. Another common occurrence is that the hair will come out, but the papilla (the hair root) will not be destroyed, resulting in the regrowth of that particular hair. Thus, depending upon the skill of the operator and the nature of the hair being treated, a single strand may have to be treated several times before it stops growing.

Coarse hairs may return three or four times, but these become finer at each regrowth, and eventually the root is so effectively destroyed that the hairs can no longer grow.

"Sittings" with the electrologist should be no longer than half an hour, during which time only a limited number of hairs (about fifty) should be removed. To avoid excessive irritation, those hairs lying close together should not be dealt with at the same time. Also, the skin and needles must be adequately sterilized to prevent infection.

In the hands of a competent, well-trained, and conscientious electrologist, the dangers and side effects are minimal. Occasionally, scarring and fine pits will develop in places formerly occupied by hairs. (One sees this more commonly on the upper lip, therefore it is best to avoid treatment on this area.) In addition, excessive pigmentation may develop, but this is rare and usually quickly disappears. Since it is impossible to predict the nature of scarring or healing in any given patient, the electrologist should try a small trial area first and check the results.

I do not recommend the small, battery-operated, do-it-your-self kits. It is virtually impossible for a person to insert a tiny needle into a hair follicle on his or her face while looking in a mirror! And when improperly used, these self-treatments can lead to irreparable scarring.

If you are contemplating electrolysis, don't expect too much. The average patient quickly tires of the experience and the cost. Because only a small percentage of hairs can be removed at one sitting, and because some regrowth of hair, even in the most skilled hands, will always recur after electrolysis, it requires firm dedication on the part of you and the operator. A severe case of excess hair (hirsutism) may require years of treatment. But despite its limitations, in selected patients electrolysis is useful and successful.

Other than these physical and mechanical methods, there are some oral medications that seem to influence and control excessive hair growth:

- The high-dose oral contraceptive pills. With their high estrogen levels, these suppress the amount of androgens (male-type hormone) in the ovaries, and act to slow down this objectionable hair production.
- Cimetidine (Tagamet)—a drug used for stomach ulcers. This drug affects male hormone production and also checks excess hair growth.
- Spironolactone—a medication used for high blood pressure. This also works as an anti-androgen, and by suppressing androgenic activity in the skin, inhibits the growth of unwanted hair.
- Dexamethasone—a cortisone-like drug. This drug suppresses the adrenal gland, and some doctors consider this to be the best treatment for hypertrichosis.

These oral medications are still in the experimental stages. Your dermatologist can give you further information about them.

COSMETICS

How you look influences how you feel—physically and emotionally. Physical beauty has always played a significant role in the way people have valued themselves and in the way they have been valued by others. We are programmed to believe that what is beautiful is also good and true. As a result, those who look neat, well-groomed, and appealing to the eye are usually more socially successful and happier than those who do not.

The use of cosmetics is one of the most common methods of achieving a particular image. Put simply, a cosmetic is "an article to be rubbed in, poured, sprinkled or sprayed on, introduced into, or otherwise applied to the human body or any part thereof for cleansing, beautifying, promoting attractiveness, or altering the appearance."

The use of cosmetics to adorn our skin and enhance our appearance goes back to the beginning of time. Skillfully used, cosmetics can change your appearance by adding color, texture, form, and shine. They can add a healthy glow to disguise winter pallor and ashiness, and camouflage minor blemishes and defects. For many women, cosmetics also help build self-confidence and self-esteem.

Cosmetic products, formerly used by only the wealthy, are now available to everyone. What cosmetics you should use is easy: whatever you like, whatever you can afford, and whatever doesn't cause any adverse reactions or side effects as itchiness, oiliness, or pimples. If you like the look, the feel, the smell, and the price, use it!

There are some general guidelines, however, to help you be a better cosmetics consumer:

- The most expensive cosmetic is not necessarily the best for you. What you pay for when you buy expensive cosmetics is fragrance, the designer's name, the cost of advertising, and fancy packaging. The expensive products, however, often have greater esthetic and psychological advantage for the buyer who feels that the more costly the better. It is more chic and "status-y," it stresses exclusivity, it has more snob appeal, and it gives the buyer a feeling of well-being. But remember, the active and useful ingredients in all cosmetics are relatively inexpensive and pretty much the same.
- Don't be sucked in by the hype that a cosmetic is "pH-balanced," "dermatologist-tested," and "hypo-allergenic." They all are! And as far as "natural" and "organic," these are meaningless terms intended to impress and confuse you.
- There are no so-called moisturizers or creams that can restore elasticity to damaged skin. And they do not slow down aging. Most moisturizers cause blackheads and white-heads!
- The best cosmetics are those that are oil-free and water based.

COSMETIC SAFETY

If used and stored properly, almost all cosmetics, except mascara which has a "life expectancy" of only three or four months, can last for about one year. Old cosmetics are risky to use and will never give you the proper results. Homemade cosmetics present problems with bacterial contamination.

If your make-up has changed color or odor, dried out, or separated, get rid of it—the chances are that it's contaminated or has outlived its usefulness.

COSMETIC DO'S

- Before you purchase an expensive cosmetic, ask for a sample to try at home.
- Keep the lids and caps of jars, bottles, and tubes tightly closed when not in use.
- Keep your jars, bottles, and tubes scrupulously clean, and store them in well-ventilated places away from excessive heat and cold.
- Clean all your sponges and cosmetic brushes frequently with a mild soap and water.
- Keep your eye pencils clean and freshen them up periodically by sharpening them.
- Change your powder puffs often.
- Always remove your makeup before going to bed.
- Check the expiration date on mascara and other cosmetics.
- Discard your mascara after three or four months or earlier, if the odor or color has changed. Mascara has a much higher risk of bacterial contamination than other cosmetics. After using mascara, always wipe the brush off with a clean, dry facial tissue.
- If you have a skin or eye infection, your cosmetics can easily become contaminated. Discard any you may have been using, and don't use any cosmetics until your problem has cleared up.

COSMETIC DON'T'S

- Never use anyone else's cosmetics and never lend yours to anyone. Swapping cosmetics can lead to contamination and can spread infection.
- Never use those so-called "tester" cosmetics from the cosmetic counters. Tester lipsticks can spread the herpes virus and other tester products can spread infection to the skin and eyes.
- Never put makeup on an unwashed face. Use a mild, gentle soap before applying any cosmetic. And do not use deodorant soaps on your face. They leave an irritating residue on the skin.
- Don't put makeup on first thing in the morning. Let the puffiness of your face disappear first.

- Never apply any eye makeup while in a moving vehicle.
- If you wear contact lenses, don't use mascara with fibers.
- Never add anything to your cosmetics. Water and other liquids encourage bacterial growth.
- Avoid cosmetics that contain fragrances.
- And never use any cosmetic that has vitamin E in it! It can only cause allergic rashes on your skin.

EAR PIERCING

'Ear ye! 'Ear ye! Pierced ears are back in vogue, and many teenagers, as well as adult women, are having it done.

And one of the latest fads, eerie, in a way, is that some young women are having each ear pierced in three or four different places and wear as many as six or eight earrings at one time.

It may come as a surprise to many, but pierced earrings were common ornaments of men in England up to the seventeenth century! And it was common in the U.S. Navy up to about fifty years ago. There has been a recent revival of this custom in young men who wear single earrings in their left ears.

Yet, harmless as the custom may seem, it isn't something that should be done casually by friends, relatives, or other unskilled individuals. The ear piercing procedure itself takes only a few moments, and is relatively painless, but it is best performed by a physician who is aware of proper sterile technique as well as some of the minor hazards that may accompany it.

People with certain diseases, such as those with a history of eczema, rheumatic fever, certain blood disorders, impetigo, and cystic type of acne, and allergies to metals, should not have their ears pierced.

The American Medical Association has warned the public of some of the complications of ear piercings, particularly when done under unsterile conditions. These include hepatitis and other internal infections (in rare cases leading to death), excessive bleeding which may form a blood tumor, raised scars (keloids), which can occur in susceptible people, and allergies to the metal (usually nickel) in the earrings.

Nickel is a powerful sensitizer, especially in contact with broken skin. Almost all earrings contain nickel. Many people believe that their 14-carat or 18-carat gold earrings are safe to use in pierced ears. Not so! The 14-carat gold jewelry has 14 parts gold and 10 parts nickel; the 18-carat gold jewelry has 18 parts gold and 6 parts nickel—enough nickel to cause and prolong allergies. As a result, there has been a "rash" of skin allergies on earlobes which resemble infection. For the most part this reaction is merely an inflammation. Occasionally, however, certain bacteria multiply on the raw, broken skin, resulting in a true infection with weeping, oozing, and crusting. If this occurs, you must consult your doctor.

To prevent this type of allergy, purchase trainer earrings made of surgical stainless steel. In addition to being made of stainless steel, these trainer earrings should be the "post" type. I do not recommend hoops or wires until at least three months after the ear-piercing procedure.

Should you have it done? If you are healthy, if you plan to have your ears pierced in a clean and sterile manner by a physician, if you do not have a history of being allergic to metals, and if you have no raised scars on your skin, the chances are that you will have no complications following your ear piercing.

Here are some other hints to help prevent infection:

- After having your ears pierced, wear the same earrings continuously for at least six weeks.
- Gently wash the front and back of your earlobes with soap and water at least twice daily. (Do not use alcohol to clean these areas, as the alcohol may dissolve or in some way react with the glue that cements the ball to the post.)
- Twirl (turn) the earrings several complete revolutions two or three times daily.

Some amount of redness and tenderness is normal after ear-piercing. If you experience any unusual pain, swelling, or discharge, call the physician who did the procedure.

COSMETIC PROBLEMS

WRINKLES

Wrinkles—those bitter reminders of the aging process—are a natural phenomenon that occurs in all of us.

As we get on in years, the skin, for a number of reasons, begins to lose its elasticity, its flexibility, and its resiliency. It becomes thinner, fine lines develop, and then, horror of horrors, wrinkles.

What really happens to our skin as we grow older? The sweat glands and oil glands, which for many years have provided moisture and lubrication to the skin, get weary, work less, and diminish in size and number. The greater portion of the oils that have made the skin smooth and supple, as well as the fluid from the sweat glands that have kept the cells plumped up and rounded, have for the most part disappeared, leaving the surface dry and cracked.

The fibers that support the skin begin to lose their strength and elasticity. Remember the old elevated trains? Just imagine that the pillars, the structures supporting the tracks, suddenly begin to bend, break, or crumble. What happens to the train and tracks? All fall down. That's basically what happens to the skin.

The supporting collagen and elastic fibers deteriorate, and the skin begins to sag over the weakened and broken understructure.

There is also a reduction in the supply of beneficial hormones delivered to the skin cells. As a result, the fat pads in the skin begin to shrink, and certain fibers, which attach the skin to the muscles, relax and become weak, causing sagging and wrinkles.

Another type of aging skin is photoaging, a type of skin change that is due almost exclusively to sun exposure. Photoaged skin is wrinkled, yellowish, rough, lax, and leathery and has spotty pigmentation and fine veins over the cheeks and nose. "Normal" aged skin, due to heredity and the aging process, is thinner, and there is loss of elasticity and a deepening of the normal expression lines.

How much you wrinkle and at what age are influenced by other factors as well:

- Hereditary factors play a major role in the production of wrinkles. People with thin skin, the Irish and Scottish, for example, age more rapidly than "thick-skinned" individuals. Black people rarely, if ever, develop wrinkles unless they have been exposed to the sun for a lifetime.
- Exaggerated facial expressions—excessive laughing and frowning, and rough massages and facial exercises—also weaken the elastic fibers and lead to premature wrinkling such as horizontal lines of the forehead, "crow's feet" about the eyes, "laugh lines," and others. There is an old witticism that contends that "the woman who never smiles never develops wrinkles!"
- Sudden weight loss, due to diet or disease, also contributes to lines and wrinkles. After having been stretched out of shape for many years, the skin is unable to retract and so begins to hang in folds. This is comparable to what happens to a person's clothes after he or she loses a great deal of weight. They become loose, baggy, and begin to rumple. And, as our bones and fat and muscles shrink, the skin around them becomes loose and baggy.
- Excessive smoking appears to be a contributing factor in the formation of wrinkles. Did you ever notice how smokers screw up their faces to prevent smoke from getting in their eyes? This, coupled with a decrease in the circulation of blood to the facial skin, results in premature lines and wrinkles.

- Exposure to the elements—heat, cold, wind, and especially sunlight—hastens and aggravates the natural aging process. You'll note that the skin of the buttocks shows none of the degenerative and aging changes that we observe on the skin exposed to the sun—the face, neck, hands, and forearms. The covered portions of your body are young; your sun-exposed parts are old.
- Excessive washing and scrubbing, especially with harsh soaps and very hot water, contribute to breakage of the elastic fibers and tend to dissolve the essential oils that help nourish the skin.

Aging and wrinkling vary from person to person, so there is no hard and fast rule to pinpoint the exact decade when a person will begin to experience these hallmarks of decline. As a rule, however, in the forties and fifties, there is a progressive shrinking of body substance—bone, fat, muscle, and fluid—but *not* of the skin. This loss of tissue volume, coupled with the weakening of the elasticity of the skin, leads to sagging.

Sagging occurs first where the skin is thinnest—the eyelids, neck, and jaw lines. Jowls develop, the neck becomes creased, lines begin to radiate from the mouth, and "crow's feet" and "bags" develop about the eyes. All this is a result of too much facial skin to cover the diminished amount of underlying tissue.

Can we do anything about wrinkles? Yes, but there are no types of cosmetic creams, potions, facial masks, exercises, acupuncture, laser treatments, injections of fetal cells, wrinkle ironing, or massages that can flatten out or permanently erase lines and wrinkles.

Mink oil, turtle oil, placenta extract and other expensive rejuvenating creams, "wrinkle creams," and facial masks do nothing more than offer temporary relief from dryness by lubricating and softening the roughened, weather-beaten skin. Likewise, those facial saunas and the "electric needle" treatments have no lasting effect on dryness, lines, or wrinkles.

Masks, saunas, and the like can provide some psychological benefits, but let's not fool ourselves—their permanent effect on the skin is zero. They cannot prevent, postpone or minimize the effects of the aging process. However, they probably won't harm you either. So if they make you feel good, enjoy them!

The only procedures that will improve lines and wrinkles are forms of cosmetic surgery and the Zyderm Collagen Implant described on page 132. "Face-lifts" by plastic surgeons (and some dermatologists) can smooth the skin of the cheeks and forehead, eliminate the "bags" about the eyes, and erase the loose, flabby skin of the neck.

A word about Retin-A. Retin-A is a prescription product that may help retard the effects of aging skin that are due to sun exposure (photoaging). While no one knows how this product works, some dermatologists think that it stimulates fresh collagen in the lower layers of the skin. The following is information I give to my patients who request Retin-A:

THE USE OF RETIN-A FOR PHOTOAGED SKIN

Retin-A is a product that *may* slow down the effects of the aging of the skin due to sun exposure. This is called "photoaged skin." Photoaged skin is wrinkled, yellowish, rough, lax, and leathery and has spotty pigmentation and fine veins over the cheeks and nose.

"Normally" aged skin, due to heredity and the aging process, is thinner, there is loss of elasticity, and there is deepening of the normal expression lines. Retin-A is *not* effective for the wrinkles of this type of skin.

If you use Retin-A, you must use it for at least 6 months before you *may* begin to see any favorable results.

DIRECTIONS FOR USE

At night:

Wash with a mild soap or cleanser (such as *Cetaphil Lotion*) and dry your skin gently.
Wait 20-30 minutes before applying the *Retin*-A.
Use an amount no larger than a small pea for entire face.
Apply to affected areas.
Smooth into skin gently; avoid mouth, nostrils, and eyes.
Next morning:
Wash off with a mild soap or *Cetaphil Lotion*, and apply a moisturizer. You may use makeup.

Some of the side effects you may experience are:

Burning	Tingling
Irritation	Dryness

Swelling	Hives
Itching	Patchy redness
Scaling	Crusting

If any of these develop and are bothersome to you, discontinue the Retin-A for a few days and then resume it every second or third night. There is no guarantee that your wrinkles will improve with this treatment.

If you are using Retin-A, avoid harsh soaps, scrubs, and granular cleansers, and do not wax on the areas where the Retin-A has been applied. Avoid sun exposure. If you have to be in the sun for any period of time, always use a sunscreen with an SPF of at least 15. PreSun 29 is a good choice.

If you use it and think that it's working, you will probably have to use it three or four times a week, forever. When you stop, the fine lines will probably reappear.

Good luck!

There are some things you can do to forestall the wrinkling process:

- Avoid the sun! I cannot stress this enough. In otherwise healthy people, sun exposure is the principal cause not only of wrinkles, aging skin, and other degenerative changes, but of skin cancers.
- Avoid extremes of heat and cold, and protect your face against the wind and rain and snow.
- Wash your face with a gentle soap and avoid excessively hot water and harsh cleansers.
- Do not lose and gain weight, off again, on again like a yo-yo. The constant expansion and contraction of the skin will only tire out the elastic fibers.
- No facial exercises or isometrics. These, when overdone, can cause a breakdown of the elastic fibers and the collagen in the skin.
- And cut down on smoking.

If you already have wrinkles, and if they are causing you great anguish, your only other options are cosmetic surgery or a collagen implant. If you can afford it, the rewards can be great, but only you can decide whether you want to alter nature—or let it take its course.

PORES

Show me a person who claims to have the "largest facial pores in the world," and I'll show you someone who owns at least one magnifying mirror!

Skin pores are the openings of hair follicles, oil glands, and sweat glands. Because they are inherited, you cannot change their size, no matter what the cosmetic firms tell you.

It is true that certain conditions may make pores "appear" larger or smaller. Oily skin and severe acne, for example, may widen the oil ducts to create the "large pore" appearance. And pores may be more apparent on the nose, cheeks, and chin where there is the greatest concentration of oil glands. Repeated squeezing of blackheads and pimples may also lead to permanently widened pores, some of which may actually be tiny, pitted scars.

Other conditions can make your pores look smaller temporarily. For instance, note what happens to your pores when you get a sunburn. They become considerably smaller due to the inflammation and swelling around the pores. Once the inflammation has subsided, the pores will return to their original appearance. Pinching or gently slapping the skin of the cheeks to make them pink has a similar, temporary pore-shrinking effect.

There is *no* scientific evidence to support the fact that pores can be made to open and close, as many advertisements would lead you to believe. Certain astringents containing acetone and alcohol, as well as various facial masks, however, can produce a temporary "shrinking" effect. These products help remove excess oil from the skin surface which makes the skin feel cool and tight. A possible explanation of this phenomenon is that the astringent or mask acts as an irritant on the skin surface. This irritation causes swelling around the pore, thus making the opening appear smaller and shrunken. Any shrinkage, however, is so insignificant and so short-lived that the time, effort, and cost involved are usually not worth the outcome.

Similarly, hot baths, hot showers, and hot packs followed by cold baths, cold showers, and cold packs do absolutely nothing to the size of the pores. The only effect this "hot-cold" theory has is to make one feel that something, a tightening, a contraction, a shriveling, whatever, is actually going on in the pores. If, however, it makes you feel good, do it! It cannot do any harm.

For those of you who think your facial pores are the largest, the ugliest, and the most noticeable, do the following:

- Wash your face thoroughly with soap and water three times a day to prevent oils from accumulating, clogging up, and distending the pores.
- Use a good, commercial astringent or face mask that makes you and your skin feel good.
- Use only oil-free and water-based cosmetics and moisturizers.
- And throw away your magnifying mirrors.

CELLULITE

A few years ago, a bestseller on the subject referred to cellulite (pronounced cell-you-leet) as a "household word in Europe." It describes the "lumps, bumps, and bulges" that do not disappear with simple diet and exercise. What the book doesn't say is that cellulite affects practically every female, of every age.

Cellulite is an invented disease. It is a "normal abnormality" that has tortured European women for many decades. The word cellulite was apparently coined at the turn of the century in European salons to describe the waffled-looking fat on women's buttocks and upper thighs. The proponents of this nondisease, seeking new markets for their advertising and useless remedies, have flooded the American market with their "miracle" products and their fraudulent claims.

To find out what cellulite looks like, make this pinch test. With your palms about four inches apart, press and squeeze together the outer part of your upper thigh. If the skin ripples and looks like a mattress, it means you have cellulite. It also probably means that you are a woman!

In a scientific investigation of almost a thousand women, this mattress-like phenomenon occurred in practically all of them. Cellulite is not found in men who have the normal amount of male hormones (androgens). It is, however, found in men who have an androgen deficiency due to hormonal disease.

Cellulite, really a fancy name for plain fat, is a sex-typical feature of women's skin and is NOT a sign of disease. It is most common on the buttocks and thighs but can also occur on the lower part of the abdomen, the upper portions of the arms, and elsewhere. Contrary to reports in nonmedical literature, cellulite is not painful, nor is it due to illness, miniskirts, or birth control pills.

What do hormones have to do with cellulite, and why do only women have it? The following is a simplified, non-technical explanation:

The reason why women have cellulite is that their skin is much thinner than that of men. As women get older, this thin skin becomes even thinner and looser, and clusters of fat cells begin to replace this lost skin. It is these fatty clusters, high up in the skin, that are responsible for the mattress-like phenomenon and the feel of cellulite.

What can you do about cellulite? The paperback bestsellers, advertisements, and commercials would have you believe that diet, proper bowel function, breathing exercises, relaxation, yoga, massage, enzyme injections, liposuction, low power laser beams, iontophoresis, "mesotherapy," or the heralded "rice treatment" can eliminate this mark of womanhood. Don't believe them. Imagine pounding or massaging a glob of chicken fat. As hard or as long as you pound or massage it, nothing is going to turn it into anything other than fat!

The best way to prevent excessive cellulite is to avoid becoming overweight. If you are overweight, slow and progressive weight loss and exercising to improve muscle tone in the buttocks and thighs may help reduce cellulite. Female athletes, by the way, show little or no cellulite. According to one of the directors of the American Medical Association's personal and public health policy, the only way to avoid cellulite altogether is to "choose a different set of grandparents, stay physically fit throughout your life, and don't be a female"!

It seems a pity that what was once depicted as "ideal" (plump figures) by such famous artists as Botticelli, Rubens, and Goya is no longer considered chic or desirable.

SCARS

Almost everyone has at least one scar—from a vaccination, cut or laceration, burn, acne, boil, chicken pox, shingles, or surgical procedures.

Scars are permanent. Some hucksters would have you believe they have "proven" products that will flatten out or eliminate scars. Don't believe them! Massaging scars with creams and potions containing such magical ingredients as turtle oil, placenta extract, cocoa butter, or vitamin E is useless and expensive.

Certain medical procedures, however, can make scars less conspicuous. These include dermabrasion (skin planing), treating them with various acids (chemical peels), and, for more serious scars, plastic surgery.

A new method is being used by dermatologists to treat certain types of scars and defects resulting from scarring diseases such as chicken pox and acne, birth defects, injury, and depressions left after surgery. This procedure is the Zyderm Collagen Implant, and it has been tested in thousands of patients in the past few years.

Collagen is the generic name for a family of proteins which are the major fibrous component of skin, tendons, ligaments, cartilage, and bone. Accounting for about one third of the total human protein, it acts as the so-called glue of the bodily tissues. (The name is taken from the Greek "kolla," meaning glue.) This jelly-like protein complex is responsible for the smooth, pliable texture of the skin and gives the skin its proper tone, resilience, and elasticity.

In the Zyderm Collagen Implant, a physician uses a fine-gauge needle to inject collagen directly into depressed or scarred areas of the skin, areas where the original collagen has been lost or destroyed. The implant fills in lines, crags, and depressions, thus raising the skin to the level of surrounding tissues.

Once injected, the implant becomes stationary, and takes on the same texture as normal skin. What is particularly remarkable is that the body accepts this implanted collagen. In fact, it appears that cells and blood vessels actually grow into the implant, making it a living part of the skin.

The number of treatment sessions, and the success of the results, will vary with the size, depth, and nature of the depression or scar. Hardened scars may require several injections to soften the tissue so that subsequent injections can correct it. And occasional "touch-up" implantations may be necessary to maintain the correction.

Adverse reactions to Zyderm are rare. To determine if you are sensitive to the implant material, your dermatologist will administer a test implantation in your forearm. You will be asked to watch the site for four weeks for any signs of sensitivity.

Very deep scars, such as those resulting from severe acne, chicken pox, and other viral infections, do not respond well to the Zyderm Implant. But for many patients this implantation procedure can provide a simpler, safer and less expensive alternative to plastic surgery.

STRETCH MARKS

Stretch marks are very thin scars that commonly develop when the skin is stretched for a long period of time. This stretching strains the elastic fibers in the deeper layers of the skin to the point where they cannot regain their original resiliency. In simple terms, the skin doesn't "snap back" to its original shape.

The most common sites for stretch marks are the abdomen, hips, buttocks, thighs, and breasts. They usually show up at puberty (when young girls and boys fill out very rapidly), and with obesity and pregnancy. People who do repeated and strenuous exercises, like weight-lifters and ballet dancers, often develop stretch marks as well. Less common factors include certain glandular disturbances, severe illnesses, such as scarlet fever and typhoid, and the use of salves and lotions containing strong cortisone-like preparations, when used in body folds over long periods of time.

Stretch marks are initially reddish or purple. After many months, however, the color usually fades out and these shallow scars become white.

There are *no* measures in the form of lotions, creams, or ointments that can decrease or erase these scars, so don't believe those ads that promise to get rid of them. Plastic surgeons may recommend a rather complicated surgical procedure that involves cutting away a great deal of skin, tightening up the underlying muscles, and following all this up with dermabrasion. Before you contemplate such a drastic measure, keep in mind that the only problem stretch marks cause is possibly a cosmetic one.

Two fairly simple measures you can take to prevent stretch marks are to avoid gaining too much weight and to avoid extreme tension on the skin.

KELOIDS

A keloid is an abnormal scar, a bizarre response to injury. Actually, it is an overgrowth of scar tissue. The scar tissue continues to form long after it is needed, building up extra tissue and resulting in a hard, smooth, and round lump.

Keloids are a medical mystery. We don't know what causes them. Nor can we predict when, where, and in whom they will occur, or how large they'll become. We do know that they are much more common in Asians and blacks, who have a tendency to develop keloids even after minor injuries.

If you have a keloid, don't be alarmed. The only problem it usually causes is cosmetic. In rare instances keloids also may be somewhat incapacitating, for example, if they develop across joints.

If the keloid is small and inconspicuous, let it be. For larger lesions and those that are cosmetically unacceptable, your dermatologist can offer a variety of treatments, but no guarantees that they will work. Keloids are highly resistant to treatment. The type of treatment your dermatologist will try will depend upon the age, size, and location of the keloids. Older and larger keloids are much more difficult to treat.

Treatment methods include injecting a cortisone-like substance directly into the keloid; removing the keloid surgically and following it up with the same cortisone injections (surgical excision alone will only make the keloid recur, and possibly even larger than the original lesion); treating it with X-rays; and freezing the area with liquid nitrogen or dry ice. Good results for stubborn keloids are being reported using the carbon dioxide laser. A new approach, the administration of bacterial collagenase, is being tried with moderate success in stubborn keloids.

SWEAT

All normal, healthy people sweat. Some more, some less. And all healthy people smell when they sweat. This, too, is normal.

Sweat is important in regulating your body temperature. Despite enormous changes in the temperature of our external environment, be it tropical or sub-zero, your internal body temperature remains fairly constant.

When you are exposed to excessive heat, the sweat glands pour out their watery secretion (sweat) and carry out the vital task of cooling your body. This thermoregulatory mechanism has allowed us to adapt to the hottest climates.

Sweat is composed of the secretion of two types of glands: the 2 million eccrine glands distributed over the entire body; and the localized apocrine glands, which are restricted primarily to the armpits, the anogenital region, and the nipples. The growth of the apocrine glands is regulated by a hormone that begins to form about the time of puberty and decreases markedly in old age. (This is why children under the age of twelve and elderly people do not suffer from "body odor.") These apocrine glands become active after puberty, respond to hormonal secretions, and are stimulated by emotional factors such as stress and sexual excitement.

135

Sweat itself is essentially odorless. Most of the odor is due to the action of various bacteria on the milky secretion of the apocrine sweat glands. These bacteria are most active in moist and warm environments, particularly hairy armpits.

Sweat from body regions devoid of apocrine glands can also have an unpleasant odor. For example, the odor of certain aromatic foods and spices (such as garlic and onions) are secreted in eccrine sweat. And eccrine sweat from prolonged exercising can cause an unpleasant odor due to bacterial action on the soft, wet skin. This is the most common cause of foot odor.

Normally, we lose about two quarts of liquid through perspiration each day. Perspiration is not under voluntary control. You cannot decide when you want to perspire and you cannot tell yourself to stop this mechanism. Emotional and environmental factors (heat) influence the degree of sweating, especially over the palms, soles, armpits, and forehead. Doctors believe that cigarette smoking may also be responsible for excessive perspiration. You can, however, "harness" this mechanism somewhat by using antiperspirants and deodorants.

Antiperspirants are compounds which reduce the volume of perspiration. Deodorants are products used to mask, diminish, or prevent perspiration odor.

ANTIPERSPIRANTS

Antiperspirants are sold as pads, creams, sprays, lotions, powders, liquids, and roll-ons. We don't know for certain how antiperspirants act, but we believe that they reduce perspiration by strictly mechanical means. Made up almost exclusively of aluminum salts, they act by either shrinking the pores, blocking the openings of the pores, or causing the sweat to be reabsorbed below the skin's surface.

No antiperspirant completely stops the flow of perspiration. And since the secretion of sweat is an essential function of the skin for temperature regulation and water metabolism, it would not be desirable if it did.

Antiperspirants should be used daily, as it takes two weeks to build up maximum protection. For best results, apply to clean skin, but not immediately after shaving. Roll-ons and creams usually give greater protection than aerosols, but the choice of one type over another is a matter of personal preference—the ease of application, lack of messiness, the absence of burning or stinging, and which TV commercial appeals to you. In cases of excessive perspiration, there is a prescription solution called Drysol, which, when used as directed, is remarkably effective in reducing the amount of underarm sweating.

DEODORANTS

Deodorants are available as powders, creams, sticks, pads, roll-ons, soaps, or sprays, and are effective for a few hours to several days. They do not in any way affect the flow of perspiration. Unlike the perfumes, colognes, and toilet waters of a previous era which merely masked perspiration odor, these products use antibacterial agents, such as neomycin, triclosan (found in certain deodorant soaps), and other bacteria-destroying chemicals, to reduce or eliminate the offending bacteria.

Some people are allergic to the popular, commercial deodorant preparations. If so, try any of the so-called hypoallergenic products.

Deodorants that do not claim to check perspiration are classified as cosmetics. If the same preparation is labeled an "antiperspirant," it becomes a drug, as it alleges to change a bodily function.

In addition to antiperspirants and deodorants, there are several general measures you can take to prevent body odor:

- Bathe frequently. Nothing beats personal cleanliness for eliminating odors.
- Keep your clothing clean. Clothing collects not only the odors but the germs responsible for them.
- Wear only cotton shirts and blouses. Polyester fibers do not "breathe," and they often retain odor even after laundering.
- Shave your armpits regularly. Bacteria *love* armpits.
- Avoid garlic, onions, and asparagus. These can produce offensive odors, especially in the summertime.
- Cut down on caffeine (coffee, tea, and cola drinks) which stimulates sweat gland activity.
- For excessive perspiration and perspiration odor of the feet, try the "tea-bag remedy" described on page 214.

Is it difficult to get rid of perspiration odor? No sweat!

PIGMENT DISORDERS

Normal skin color, an important part of everyone's life, is dependent upon the amount and size of certain pigment granules in the upper layers of the skin. This basic skin color is determined at birth and cannot be altered.

All human skin contains three important pigments:

1. Melanin—this black pigment in your skin is produced by special pigment cells called melanocytes. All of us, black, yellow, red, and white people, *have the same number of these melanocytes in our skin* (approximately 60,000 per square inch).

Then why aren't we all black?

Racial and ethnic variations in skin color depend on the size and shape of these melanocytes, the amount of melanin they produce, the speed at which the pigment is formed, the manner in which this pigment is concentrated in the skin, and the color of the melanin, which can vary from light tan to black.

Melanin is produced in the skin as small, insoluble granules. Where there are no melanin granules, the skin is white; the more

138

melanin granules, the darker the skin. The variations in your particular skin color, tan, brown, black, will depend upon the concentration of these granules in your epidermis.

In black people, melanin production is evenly distributed, producing uniform skin color. In redheads, and in some blonds with blue eyes, melanin is produced in clumps, resulting in splotchy pigmentation, freckles.

Freckles, probably the most common pigmentary alteration in the skin, first appear at about the age of six as flat, light-brown, pigmented spots over sun-exposed skin. During the summer, they have a tendency to increase in number, size, and darkness.

The depth of the melanin granules will also affect the color of your skin—the deeper the granules, the more your skin will take on a bluish cast.

1. Hemoglobin—this pigment is responsible for giving red blood cells their color. If you are anemic, your skin will be pale. If you have too much hemoglobin, your skin will take on a ruddy complexion.
2. Carotene—this pigment, which gives your skin a yellowish cast, comes from outside the body, and is dependent upon what you eat. A diet consisting of large amounts of oranges, carrots, and squash can be responsible for an orange-yellow coloring of the skin.

EXCESSIVE PIGMENTATION

The most common cause of excessive pigmentation is an increased stimulation in the production of melanin due to certain hormonal changes, sun exposure, or a combination of both. This condition, called melasma, appears as a dark, splotchy, brownish pigmentation on the face that develops slowly and fades with time. It usually affects women, but occasionally is seen in young men who use aftershave lotions, scented soaps, and other toiletries.

Melasma is especially common in young white women, who often develop this blotchiness on their foreheads, cheeks, and mustache areas. It occurs frequently during pregnancy and is more common in brunettes than in blonds. Often called "the mask of pregnancy," melasma is more pronounced in summer, due to sun exposure, and usually fades a few months after delivery. Repeated pregnancies, however, often increase the intensity of this pigmentation.

Melasma also occurs as a side effect of taking the higher-dose birth control pills. It may also be noted in apparently healthy, normal, nonpregnant women due to some mild and harmless hormonal imbalance.

Sun exposure, following the use of deodorant soaps, scented toiletries, and various cosmetics, can also produce this mottled pigmentation. This is what we call a phototoxic reaction; it is due to ultraviolet radiation being absorbed by the chemical substance (perfume, cologne, and other types of fragrance) on the skin. This pigmentation often extends down to the sun-exposed areas of the neck and may be more pronounced on the left side of the forehead, face, and neck due to sun exposure while driving a car.

Excess pigmentation can also be triggered by injury to the skin (burns, abrasions, bruises), by inflammatory disorders of the skin particularly in dark-skinned people (acne, eczema, contact dermatitis, pityriasis rosea, lichen planus), by X-rays, and by heat.

TREATING EXCESSIVE PIGMENTATION

How can you treat excessive pigmentation of the skin?

Above all, protect those pigmented areas from sunlight by using a "high-powered" sunscreen (PreSun 39).

Protect the areas from irritation—no strong soaps, no abrasive cleansers, no Buf-Pufs, no loofah pads. Use only a mild, gentle soap for washing.

Try one of the over-the-counter bleaching creams (*Porcelana, Esoterica, Artra, Eldoquin*) and use only as directed. Ironically, some of these can cause further pigmentation if they are too strong for your particular skin.

A good home remedy that often works is fresh lemon juice. Cut a fresh lemon in half and squeeze the juice into a small dish. With a Q-Tip or cotton ball, gently rub the patches twice daily.

If these don't work, try *Hytone Cream* 0.5% once or twice daily.

With any local, over-the-counter product, you must remember to be patient. It may take months before you notice any appreciable fading. Occasionally, even without treatment, those dark areas may eventually fade away.

If you believe that your pigmentation is a result of taking birth control pills, try to switch to a lower-dose type with the approval of your doctor or, if possible, stop them altogether.

If none of these treatments work, your dermatologist can try a variety of methods to eliminate these pigmented areas:

- Freezing them off gently with liquid nitrogen
- Applying either phenol or trichloroacetic acid
- Prescribing topical retinoic acid (Retin-A) along with a strong hydroquinone cream
- Desiccating them lightly with an electric needle

If your condition does not respond to any type of treatment, or while waiting for the dark areas to disappear, you can mask them with a cover-up such as Covermark or Dermablend.

Above all, try to be patient.

VITILIGO—LOSS OF PIGMENTATION

Vitiligo is a mysterious malady characterized by a gradual or rapid loss of pigment, or skin color. It affects about one out of every hundred people and is more common among younger individuals. Approximately half the people who develop this ailment suffer some pigment loss before the age of twenty.

No one knows what triggers this strange condition. The most fashionable theory claims that it is one of the autoimmune disorders in which the body attacks and destroys its own tissues—in this case the pigment-producing cells. We *do* know that it results from a decrease or loss of the normal cells (melanocytes) which are responsible for the production of pigment (melanin) in the skin. If the melanocytes are unable to produce melanin, or if their number decreases, white, sharply-bordered patches of different shapes and sizes will develop on otherwise normal skin.

Vitiligo can occur on any portion of the skin surface where pigment cells are present, but more commonly involves the exposed parts—the face, neck, and backs of the hands. There is no way to predict how much pigment a person will lose. In severe cases the loss of pigment can extend over the entire body. The hairs in these depigmented patches also turn white. When the pigment returns, it returns first in and around these hairs.

The pattern of vitiligo is unclear, although the condition appears to run in families. Most of the people afflicted are in good health. Occasionally, however, vitiligo occurs in association with such conditions as pernicious anemia, thyroid disease, diabetes, and disorders of the adrenal glands. Some cases follow sunburn or severe emotional stress. If you do have this cosmetic blight called vitiligo, be assured that it is not a sign of cancer.

While this pigmentary failure can occur in all races, the cosmetic, as well as the psychological, implications are considerably greater for those with darker skins. Vitiligo is a dramatic process in dark-skinned people, often causing profound despair. In India, for example, vitiligo is considered by the populace to be a sure sign of leprosy. Nehru, realizing the myths and superstitions surrounding this perfectly benign condition, often remarked that a treatment for vitiligo was as important for his people as the treatment for leprosy and tuberculosis.

Vitiligo is usually a progressive and relentless disease, and rarely do people with the condition regain their color spontaneously. There may be a long period of time where the depigmented patches remain about the same and very often an emotional upset, infection, or illness may activate the process again with the old spots getting larger and new spots developing.

Unfortunately, there is no reliable method of regaining lost pigment. Current therapy consists of taking a special pill (a psoralen) and exposing the affected skin to sunlight or long-wave ultraviolet radiation (UVA). This form of therapy, commonly called the PUVA treatment (from *P*soralen *U*ltra*V*iolet *A*), is similar to the way dermatologists treat extensive psoriasis. But even this procedure may have to be carried out for a number of months or years before any noticeable repigmentation occurs.

Not everyone is a good candidate for repigmentation. Ideally, the person should meet the following criteria:

- A person should be in good health. Pregnant women should not be treated.
- For people over twenty years of age, pigment loss should be less than five years.
- One should be at least ten years old.
- Because treatment is a long process, the person must be committed to it and have the time to follow through.

The prognosis for vitiligo is discouraging at best. Whatever the treatment, only about one in five patients responds at all, and relapses are the rule. When the involved loss of pigment is in small patches, certain types of makeup (such as Covermark or Dermablend) and "stains" (such as Dy-O-Derm Lotion) can help camouflage the patches of vitiligo.

For more information concerning vitiligo, write to:

National Vitiligo Foundation
P.O. Box 6337
Tyler, Texas 75711
214/561-4700
Allen C. Locklin, President

NAILS

Just think: if you didn't have fingernails, how would you open your birthday presents, untie your shoelaces, button your shirt, peel off labels, or pull tacks out of bulletin boards? A variety of simple, everyday tasks would be difficult or impossible without fingernails.

You couldn't pluck guitar strings, pick up coins or take off earrings. It would be pretty challenging to open flip-top cans, peel oranges, or separate Life Savers that are stuck together. And, thanks to nails, you can scratch where it itches.

Our twenty nails are pretty important, and though we neglect and abuse them, they serve us for a lifetime. And we spend more than $200 million a year to keep them beautiful and "healthy" even though our nails are actually dead.

Once the human's only tools, the function of nails has changed in the course of evolution. In lower animals, nails—as sharp claws or strong hooves—serve for protection, locomotion, climbing and eating.

Historically, nails have been a means of personal decoration. Long nails, often accented by jeweled fingertip extenders, were a mark of the leisure class in Asian cultures for many centuries.

Growing up to a foot long, they were the sign of a life of complete idleness. Even today, well-manicured nails can be a status symbol. Some salons offer gold tips and diamond studs along with the hot pink polish.

Although our nails have now become relatively weak and flat, they still serve many useful functions:

- They protect the tips of our fingers and toes from injury and foreign substances.
- They aid the fingertips in our sense of touch.
- They help us grasp small objects and use our fingers more efficiently. This is important in delicate mechanical work.
- Nails help in defense and attack.
- They are used for scratching.
- They can serve as a mirror of our general state of health. Problems with our nails can be an indication of an internal disease.

WHAT EXACTLY ARE NAILS?
Made up of a protein called keratin, nails are specialized horny extensions of our skin. This protein has a high amount of sulfur and it's the sulfur that makes the nails hard and rigid. (For added strength, nails are curved in both directions.) The keratin of our nails is similar to the keratin that makes up our hair. Nails and hair have many things in common:

- Both have their beginnings deep inside the skin.
- Both are dead, so that they can be cut or trimmed painlessly. And since they aren't living, there's nothing you can put on them to make them grow any better, faster, longer, stronger, or thicker.
- Both depend upon the body's processes and a rich blood supply for nourishment and growth.
- Both can regenerate. If you pluck a hair out of your head, it grows back normally; if you lose a nail, it usually grows back normally as well.

Nails consist of several structures: (*see Figure*)

1. *The nail plate.* This is what we mean when we refer to our "nail." It's firmly attached to the nail bed underneath.

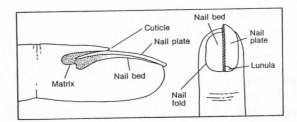

2. *The nail bed*. This network of capillaries supplies the blood and gives the pinkish color to the nail plate.

3. *The nail matrix*. This is the most important structure of our nail. Made up of living cells that produce the nail plate, it is located beneath the cuticle. If this matrix is damaged, the nail will be distorted.

4. *The lunula*. The visible part of the matrix is called the lunula or "half moon"—the small, lighter-colored arc you usually see on your thumbs and big toes. The shape of the end of your nail plate depends on the shape of your half moons.

5. *The cuticle*. The cuticle is the fold of skin at the base of the nail plate. Made up of dead cells, it seals the skin to the nail to keep foreign substances from working their way into the narrow space between the skin and the nail.

Nails will grow indefinitely if not cut or injured. They grow at different rates for everyone, depending on each person's state of health. It takes about five months for a fingernail to grow from the cuticle to the end of your fingertip. It takes longer for a thumb nail and twice as long for toenails.

Here are some other trivia to nail you with:

- Nails grow faster in summer than in winter, faster during the day than at night, faster in men than in women, and faster in children than in adults.
- Nail growth slows down as we get older, and nails tend to thicken and become irregular.
- The middle fingernail grows the fastest, and the pinkie nail the slowest.
- If you are right-handed, your nails grow faster on the right hand and vice versa.

- Nails grow faster in nail-biters, typists, and piano players, which is convenient since they use them up faster!
- They grow faster in women who are premenstrual and who are in the early stages of pregnancy.
- Starvation diets slow down the growth of nails.
- Gelatin has absolutely no value in treating nails problems.

Despite what the horror movies would make you believe, nails do not grow after death. What seems like continued nail growth is only the drying and shrinking of the soft tissues around the nail plates.

We used to believe that the hardness of nails, like bones and teeth, was the result of their calcium content. Actually, there's very little calcium in the nail plate, not enough to make a difference. So taking calcium supplements won't help soft nails.

"HEALTHY" NAILS AND NAIL CARE

Actually, there is no such thing as a healthy nail. Since the nail plate is dead, it can't really be healthy.

But you can have healthy-*looking* nails, smooth and neatly trimmed. Healthy-looking nails have no grooves, ridges or pits, and no spots or discolorations.

Nails, by nature, are hard and strong. But, like the skin and other body organs, they should be treated with gentle care.

Here are a few guidelines to help you grow and keep healthy-looking and attractive nails:

- Since nails are easier to cut when they're soft, soak them in warm water for about 30 minutes before cutting and trimming them. File them when dry.
- Don't overuse polishes, base coats and polish remover. They can cause nail problems and irritate your skin.
- Remove hangnails with clean, sharp scissors. Pulling or biting them can lead to infection.
- Treat your cuticles gently. Be careful when using cuticle-removing solutions since they can destroy tissue when left on too long. If you want to push back your cuticles, first soak your fingertips in warm water for about 20 minutes and then gently push them back using an orange stick. Remember that your cuticle is there for a purpose—to protect your nail. Tampering with it opens the door to harmful germs and

possible infection. It's a better idea just to leave your cuticles alone.

- If you wear rubber gloves, even the cotton-lined variety, always wear soft, cotton liners (Dermal gloves) inside them. When your hands are in hot water, they sweat and react with the chemicals from the rubber, plastic or vinyl in the gloves. This can cause problems for your skin and nails.
- When gardening or doing other heavy work, protect your nails by wearing canvas gloves.
- To prevent chipping, peeling and tearing, and to keep your nails flexible, moisturize them. Soak them in water for 20 minutes and then apply an emollient cream, such as Complex 15 or Candermyl cream.
- To strengthen nails, tap them—on desks, table tops and other surfaces.
- Do not use your nails as a screwdriver, can opener, pliers, or telephone dialer (not a problem with push-button phones).
- To prevent ingrown toenails, cut them straight across, so that the edges of the nail don't poke into the skin folds along the sides.

NAIL COSMETICS

Decorating the nails is a universal practice that's been around since the beginning of time. Today there are dozens of products and preparations to decorate, as well as to protect and repair the nails.

We have nail enamels, varnishes and lacquers; top coats, base coats and undercoats; nail conditioners, hardeners and whiteners; buffing creams; enamel removers and cuticle removers; cuticle creams and oils; pre-formed, plastic and gold press-on nails; sculptured and porcelain nail extenders; nail mending and nail wrapping kits.

While some of these products can make nails more resistant to damage, all of them could possibly cause irritation and allergic reactions. The dyes in nail polish can cause rashes on your eyelids, face, neck, upper chest, and even in the anal and genital areas—but almost never around your nails. The glues, resins and formaldehyde found in many nail products can irritate the nail plate and surrounding tissues and result in brittleness, discoloration, pain, lifting up of the nail, and infection.

NAIL DISORDERS

The condition of your nails, like that of your skin and hair, depends on your general health. When your body suffers from infection, disease or dietary deficiency, the growth, texture and appearance of your nails can change.

The most common nail problems are caused by fungous infections, psoriasis, lichen planus, pigmentation, and allergies to nail cosmetics.

Sudden and serious physical stress, as from a tragic accident or a major surgical operation, may dramatically change the pattern of your nail growth. This happens because nail growth is expendable, which means that your body ignores it under severe stress. The growth of your nails may slow down temporarily or stop altogether. Weeks after your health has improved, you'll be able to see transverse ridges on all your nails, showing the period when growth was interrupted.

Other changes in your nails can be a sign of illness, injury, poor nail care of other factors.

Brittle nails are nails that have lost their strength. They split, chip, crack and break off easily. Brittleness is usually due to the use of harsh household products, strong soaps and detergents, glues, cleaning solvents, furniture polish, and irritating and allergenic nail cosmetics (polish, removers, hardeners, etc.)

The weather can also cause brittleness. When the relative humidity is very low, the water content of the nail is decreased, making the nail more rigid and likely to fracture.

Finally, brittle and fragile nails can be a result of a protein deficiency, crash dieting, some illnesses and skin diseases.

Nails can also develop *ridges*. These irregular bumps can run either along the nail's length (longitudinal) or horizontally across the nail (transverse).

Longitudinal ridges are often related to an anemic condition. Transverse ridges are usually caused by an inflammation of the skin around the nail due to skin diseases such as eczema and allergic dermatitis, or sometimes by an injury which stops the growth of the nail. As mentioned earlier, ridges can also mark the onset of a severe illness, infection, prolonged fever or surgery.

Another common condition is *thickening of the nail*. This happens on the toenails when you let them grow too long or wear tight shoes that cramp their growth. Thick nails are also associated with flat feet, obesity, and fungous infections of the nails.

Pitting and stippling of the nails are caused by a defect in the growth center (matrix) of the nail. These small indentations on the nail plate are often seen in people who have psoriasis, eczema or alopecia areata.

Thinning of the nails happens with anemia, thyroid disorders and protein deficiency in crash-dieters.

Spoon-shaped depressions in the nails can be a sign of anemia, as well as thyroid and other hormonal disorders.

Separation of the nail plate from the nail bed is a common condition. Each time you clean under your nail with a fingernail file or a toothpick, you cause a tiny separation between the nail plate and the nail bed. Repeated cleanings cause a dead space to form where moisture and germs collect and grow. The nail bed becomes infected, the nail plate separates from the bed, and the color underneath the nail changes from pink to yellow, green or black, depending on which germ has set up housekeeping.

Sometimes this happens from spending a lot of time with your hands in soap and water, as well as from injury, certain drugs, fungous infections, psoriasis, and thyroid disorders.

Pigmented (discolored) nails occur for a variety of reasons. Nails can become permanently stained from heavy smoking, and working with inks, shoe polishes, dyes and chemicals. Nail injuries and tight shoes can make your nails turn black due to bleeding beneath the affected nails. For example, athletes in track and field events, joggers, tennis and racquet ball players, and dancers can develop blackened toenails from jamming their feet into the front of their shoes.

More seriously, discolored nails may be a clue to some skin or internal disease. Fungal and bacterial infections, diabetes, and certain lung, liver and kidney diseases can all change the color of your nails. So can antibiotics, anti-cancer drugs, sulfa and other medications.

White spots are often seen on the nails as a result of rough manicuring, typing, filing and nail-biting, as well as from nutritional deficiency, fungous infections, thyroid conditions, and anemia.

Nail *breakage* can occur from using the nails as handy tools. Nails are strong, but not as strong as screw drivers, can openers, and pliers.

Paronychia is an infection or inflammation around the nail folds caused by bacteria or fungous germs. It can result from a nail injury, nail-biting, and from keeping your hands in water for a long time. It's a common problem for bartenders, waitresses, and housewives (and househusbands).

TREATMENT OF NAIL DISORDERS

The treatment of nail disorders will depend upon the type of problem you have and what's causing it. Try to figure out and get rid of what you think might be responsible for the condition. Correct any general disorder or disease you may have, and eat a well-balanced diet.

For a continuing and stubborn nail problem, see your dermatologist. Remember, nails can be a mirror of other, more serious health problems.

SUN-RELATED
SKIN CONDITIONS

The suntan. The envy of friends and relatives. The bronzed lifeguard. The golden, tawny bodies on the sand. The sad truth is that suntanning is a dangerous habit with no benefit except the elusive psychological one: looking good and healthy means feeling good and healthy. Exposure to the sun is directly and ultimately responsible for the leathery look of prematurely aged skin, wrinkles, and skin cancer—all of which are irreversible. It can also cause sun-poisoning.

The serious problems caused by the sun's rays are getting worse as a result of the thinning of the ozone layer in the earth's atmosphere. The ozone layer normally gives us some protection from the sun, but due to aerosols, propellants, nitrogen oxides from nuclear explosions and supersonic transports, and chlorine from space shuttles, this protective layer has been partially depleted.

The following chapters describe the process behind sun tanning, how to suntan properly, and how to treat and prevent sun-poisoning.

SUNTANNING

Tanning is nothing more than the body's efficient, protective mechanism: a response to injury from sunlight and a way to protect us from additional injury. That "healthy-looking" tan, usually associated with good health and enviable sex appeal, is, in fact, damaged skin.

In early times, suntanned skin was associated with those who worked outdoors for a living—the peasants, the farmers, the serfs. People of means, those from the upper social classes, took pains to stay out of the sun to preserve their natural color. Medieval beauties were admired for their indoor pallor and the traditional fresh fairness of Englishwomen, a combination of genes, high humidity, and minimum sunlight, has been extolled by lovers and envied by other women.

Because the tanning mechanism is not one hundred percent efficient, repeated sun exposure allows certain wavelengths of light to penetrate this defense barrier, causing the various sun-related skin conditions.

The more subtle changes caused by the sun's rays may not be apparent for decades, but they do and will occur in every person who is foolish enough to expose himself or herself to excess. Therefore, the only good suntan is no suntan at all.

Compare the sun-exposed portions of your body—your face, hands, forearms—with those parts of your anatomy (your buttocks, for example) that are almost never exposed. Note the difference in smoothness and texture. Your buttocks are young, your hands and face are old.

For you fair-haired, fair-skinned, and blue-eyed people, tanning, if it does occur, is a slow process. You have much smaller pigment cells than your dark-haired, darker-skinned, brown-eyed neighbors. So you burn more easily and require infinitely more sun exposure to produce even a modest tan. If you are dark-skinned, on the other hand, merely a brief exposure to the sun often produces a lasting tan.

For you light-skinned people who, despite all admonition, still desire that bronzed look, here are a few rules:

Acquire your tan gradually. If you head for the beaches, the backyards, and the lake in order to soak up that first Sunday sun in June, avoid a severe and painful sunburn by limiting your first

exposure to fifteen or twenty minutes. Increase the exposure gradually by twenty or thirty minutes a day for four or five more days. The first pigment cells will then begin to show up to darken and protect the skin. From then on, you can tolerate almost any length of exposure.

If you are a redhead or a blond, you do not have adequate pigment cells to begin with. Therefore, you must be more careful and reduce the early exposure times by approximately half.

All this, however, is trial and error. Only *you* will know how much sun you can tolerate on first and subsequent exposures without causing painful sunburn.

Keep in mind that the most intense rays of the sun occur between 10 A.M. and 2 P.M. (standard time), the overhead sun being the strongest. You cannot get sunburned before 9 A.M. and after 5 P.M., at which times the sharply angulated "burn" rays have been filtered out by the atmosphere.

Also, don't let overcast skies fool you. Sunburn can occur on hazy and foggy days. And don't think that only direct exposure to the sun produces burning or tanning. Reflected rays from sand, cement, and water can also cause severe sunburn. Beach umbrellas do not offer absolute protection. And you can even get sunburned while swimming under water!

Use suntan creams and lotions. Many of the suntan preparations contain certain chemicals which selectively absorb the shorter wavelengths of sunlight that are responsible for burning. This will permit some of the longer wavelengths of light—the tanning rays—to penetrate the skin.

People are classified into various skin types depending on their levels of melanin pigmentation. And, depending upon the type of skin you have, there is a wide range of sunscreen products that are rated according to the degree of protection they can give against ultraviolet radiation. This rating is called the Sun Protection Factor (SPF).

This SPF is a guide and a numbering system to assess the efficacy of sunscreen agents. The number represents the number of times longer you can stay in the sun if you use the product than if you used nothing. A number 15, for example, will provide 15 times the user's natural skin protection.

A list of these products, with the appropriate SPF, appears on page 157.

Skin Type I: People with fair hair and fair skin or freckles are most susceptible to the sun's rays. They can develop a severe sunburn in a matter of minutes and also have a higher risk of developing skin cancers and wrinkles. If you are Skin Type I, you won't tan no matter how long you bake in the sun. Persistent sunbathing is not only futile, but downright dangerous. Always use sunscreens with a Sun Protection Factor of at least 15.

Skin Type II: These people are also fair-skinned but not as sensitive to the sun's rays as those of Type I. They usually burn and only occasionally develop a "weak" tan. Use sunscreens with an SPF of 10 to 15.

Skin Type III: This type includes people with darker skin who usually tan but sometimes burn. Use sunscreens with an SPF of 6 to 10.

Skin Type IV: These people always tan well and almost never develop sunburn. They can use sunscreens with an SPF of 2 to 6.

When using any suntanning product, follow the directions given by the manufacturer, and reapply it every two or three hours. Always reapply after swimming.

The best approach to suntanning is common sense. This large envelope we call the skin has to last a lifetime, so give it the protection it deserves.

A word about those tanning salons that have sprung up all over the country. Although advertised as using the "safer" long-wave ultraviolet rays (UVA), the lamps used in these salons are fraught with the same hazards as other forms of radiation. There are definite dangers associated with repeated exposure to UVA. In addition to the premature aging, wrinkles, and the potential for developing skin cancer, other harmful effects may include:

- Damage to the eyes, resulting in cataracts.
- Aggravation of existing skin damage caused by sun exposure.
- Aggravation of "light-sensitive" skin disorders, such as cold sores and lupus erythematosus.
- Damage to older people who already have thinner skin.
- Adverse reactions to certain soaps, toiletries, high blood pressure medications, tranquilizers, birth control pills, etc.
- Changes in the immune system and in the blood vessels in the skin.

Do your skin—and yourself—a favor: stay away from those artificial tanning rays.

A note about children's skin: since children often spend many hours playing in the sun, protecting children's skin from the sun's harmful rays is one of the most important ways to promote their long-term health. Before sun exposure, always apply a sunscreen with a SPF of at least 15 to your child's skin regardless of his or her age.

SUN-POISONING

Sun-poisoning is a nonscientific term that refers to a variety of sun-allergic responses. Light-skinned people, who have less protective skin pigment, are especially susceptible to sun-poisoning, but it can occur in anyone who is exposed to enough light. It often occurs in combination with a variety of drugs, chemicals, cosmetics, and plants.

The classic example of sun-poisoning is sunburn. We all know that redheads suffer more from the effects of the sun's rays than the rest of the population. This is because they lack enough melanin pigment (one of the main defense mechanisms against sunburn) in the skin. Black people rarely suffer from sunburn because the pigment in their epidermis (the upper layers of the skin) prevents the penetration of the sunburn rays to the sensitive, deeper layers of the skin.

If you are a susceptible person, certain common drugs you may be taking can change your normal protective response to the sun. The result can be a severe rash with blisters from just the slightest exposure to sunlight or even fluorescent lighting. Drugs most commonly involved in this type of reaction are the sulfa drugs, "relatives" of tetracycline, various tranquilizers, high blood pressure medication, birth control pills, and oral medications used for diabetes and fungous infections (ringworm). Direct contact with certain chemicals, followed by sun exposure also can cause sun-poisoning. The most common substances that cause these "sun-allergic" responses are found in deodorant bar soaps, detergents, certain suntan lotions, shampoos, "first-aid" creams, and various cosmetics and toiletries.

Even chemicals found in a variety of vegetables and fruits can cause sun-sensitive reactions. Gardeners and farmers who spend time in the sun and handle such foods as carrots, celery, parsnips, figs, and limes are especially susceptible. Sun-poisoning has also been reported as a result of using herbal shampoos followed by sun exposure.

The symptoms of sun allergy are severe itching and rash which occur a few days after the combination of the chemical substance and the light. This sensitivity can be so pronounced that a minute amount of the substance left on your skin, followed by exposure even to fluorescent light, may trigger a reaction.

The treatment for sun-poisoning is essentially the same as for any allergic dermatitis, such as poison ivy dermatitis. If your case is mild, use wet compresses or soothing baths followed by calamine lotion to relieve your symptoms. If your itching is more persistent, take an antihistamine. For any severe reaction accompanied by intense itching and blisters that weep and ooze, see your dermatologist. You may need treatment for dehydration and possible infection.

PREVENTING SUN-POISONING

Preventing sun-sensitive reactions may take a lot of trial and error to determine which drug, chemical, or plant is the culprit. Once you've discovered it, eliminate it from your routine. If the offender is a drug that is essential for your health (high blood pressure pills or antidiabetic medications for example), you'll need to stay out of the sun at all times.

If you are fair-skinned, the best way to avoid a sun-sensitive reaction is to avoid the sun. If this just isn't possible, then tan slowly and cautiously. (See guidelines on page 153)

To prevent overexposure to the sun, use a good sunscreen. Sunscreens usually contain chemicals that selectively block out or absorb all the harmful "short" ultraviolet rays, permitting some of the longer, tanning rays to get through to the skin.

Sunscreens

For Skin Type I—SPF 15 or over
PreSun 39 (Westwood)
Super Shade 25 (Plough)
Solbar Plus 15 (Person & Covey)
For Skin Type II—SPF 10 to 15
PreSun 15 (Westwood)
Sundown Sunscreen Ultra Protection Lotion 15 (Johnson & Johnson)
Coppertone Sunblock Lotion 15 (Plough)
For Skin Type III—SPF 6 to 10
PreSun 8 (Westwood)
Sundown Sunscreen Lotion 8 (Johnson & Johnson)
For Skin Type IV—SPF 2 to 6
PreSun 4 (Westwood)
Sundown Sunscreen Lotion 4 (Johnson & Johnson)

Another good, but cosmetically inelegant, sun-blocking preparation is zinc oxide paste.

To protect the delicate areas of the lips, use a "lipstick" that contains a sun-blocking agent, such as

PreSun Lip Protector SPF 15 (Westwood)
Super Shade Sunblock Stick SPF 25 (Plough)

TREATING SUN-POISONING

For an acute case of sun-poisoning with redness, itching, burning, and blisters, treat it the same as you would any acute rash.

If the condition is localized, use warm compresses with

Bluboro Powder (Herbert)

Directions are on the package. Use as open wet dressings as described on page 217.

For a widespread sunburn, take soothing baths in either of the following:

Alpha Keri Bath Oil (Westwood) or
Nutraderm Bath Oil (Owen)

Directions are on the bottles.

A good point to remember is that sun-poisoning (a burn) is similar to a fire. Just as you would use cold water to put out the fire, use wet compresses or baths to get fast relief. Never use soap during this stage.

Following the compresses or baths, use either of the following creams to help relieve the itching and permit the skin to maintain its smoothness and softness:

Hytone Cream 0.5 (Dermik)
Cort-Aid Cream (Upjohn)

Directions: Apply every 3 or 4 hours and after your bath.

For the itching that may accompany the healing stage of sun-poisoning, take either of the following antihistamines every four hours when necessary:

Chlor-Trimeton Tablets [4 mg] (Schering)
Dimetane Tablets [4 mg] (Robins)

See Directions and cautions on the label for proper dosage.

If the sunburn is painful, take aspirin every 3 or 4 hours as needed. If your sun-poisoning is severe, with a great deal of pain, huge blisters, or denuded skin, see your doctor at once.

To protect from further bouts of sun-poisoning, always use a sun protective sunscreen at least an hour *before* exposure to the sun.

ITCHING

"Scratching is one of the sweetest gratifications of nature,
and as ready at hand as any."

Montaigne

Itching, simply stated, is the urge to scratch. The medical term
for itching is pruritus. It is common, everyday experience ranging
from a simple, fleeting annoyance (a mosquito bite) to the intense,
distressing, unrelieved torment (the itch of scabies) that can result
in sleepless nights.

Why do people itch? Let me try to explain.

We know that the sensations of pain and itch are carried to the
brain by the same nerve fibers, and we know that pain and itching
points have similar distribution on the surface of the skin. We also
know that it's possible, by varying the intensity of a stimulus
(chemical, electrical, or physical) to cause either pain or itching on
a certain portion of the skin.

So, a better way of understanding this complex sensation is
thinking of an itch as a sub-threshold pain, or, better still, as a pain
that doesn't hurt.

Have you ever bruised or scraped or skinned your knee or elbow? Have you ever suffered from a moderately severe sunburn? If you have, you may remember that at first there were varying degrees of pain. When the bruise or scrape or burn began to heal, this pain was gradually transformed into an itch—a so-called "healing" itch: a desire to scratch.

Commonly experienced, unpredictable, and poorly understood, itching is the symptom that most frequently prompts a person to visit a dermatologist.

Different people experience, interpret, and tolerate itching in different degrees. If you have a high itch threshold, a transient mosquito bite or a brush with a poison ivy plant will rarely bother you. Less fortunate people will itch unmercifully at the least provocation, such as a mild allergy to nickel earrings or a simple rash from a leather watchband. No one knows why.

Many years ago scientists thought the basic cause of itching was the release of a chemical substance called histamine. We now know that itching can be caused by a breakdown of various tissue proteins, and can be precipitated by a variety of stimuli:

Chemicals: plants (poison ivy), drugs (aspirin, penicillin), foods (berries, seafood, nuts), metals (nickel, chromium), cosmetics, paints and sprays, and hundreds more.
Physical: heat, cold, pressure, and friction.
Infestations: lice, mites (scabies), insect bites and stings.
Germs: athlete's foot, cold sores, impetigo.
Skin disorders: eczema, allergy rashes, hives, lichen planus, dry skin.
Psychogenic: anxiety, tension, emotional stress.
Systemic disease: diabetes and other hormonal disorders, liver and kidney problems, malignant diseases.
Blood disorders: leukemias, Hodgkin's disease.

What do you do when you itch? You scratch.

Why does scratching relieve itching? Again, no one really knows. It may be that by scratching or rubbing you are substituting the sensation of pain for that of itching. Or, it may be that by scratching or digging with your nails you damage the nerve fibers that cause the itching. Scratching, while it may give you temporarily relief, can actually cause more harm than good. It can lead to secondary infection which may require internal antibiotic therapy.

What *should* you do when you itch?

The most important thing to do is determine, if you can, why you began to itch in the first place. If you don't have a clue, and if your itch persists, see a dermatologist. She or he will try to uncover the cause and, if possible, eliminate it. What you can do to relieve your itching depends, of course, on the cause. No single therapy is effective for all itching. In addition to providing symptomatic relief, most treatments are aimed at eliminating the underlying cause.

For symptomatic relief of mild to moderate itching—regardless of the cause—there are several over-the-counter remedies you can try:

1. Oral antihistamines, such as Dimetane, Chlor-Trimeton, or Benadryl. (Take according to the directions on the package.)
2. Hytone Cream 0.5 for localized itchy areas, or
3. Phenolated calamine lotion. Apply to the itchy areas every 3 or 4 hours.
4. If the itching is fairly generalized, take soothing baths using a therapeutic baths oil such as Alpha Keri Bath Oil.

If your itching is severe, persistent, and unrelieved by over-the-counter measures, consult with a dermatologist. It may not be a simple itch after all.

OTHER COMMON
SKIN AILMENTS

―――――――

We have already examined most of the familiar skin conditions. There are literally hundreds more. Some of the other
common and annoying disorders of the skin and mucous membranes are discussed in the following section.

CANKER SORES

Canker sores are painful ulcerations in the mouth affecting
about twenty-five percent of the population. The medical term for
this baffling condition is aphthous stomatitis—but these sores by
any other name are just as painful.

Many people confuse canker sores with cold sores. Cold sores
are caused by a virus. But we know little about what causes canker
sores and even less about what cures them. Nor do we know what
prevents them. We *do* know that they are not contagious, they are
more common in women, they are not hereditary, and they do not
cause cancer.

Canker sores develop as small blisters in the mouth, singly or
in groups, which usually go unnoticed. These blisters break, and

small, round, shallow ulcers develop. The ulcers gradually enlarge and become yellow and shiny with bright red borders. They can be exquisitely tender and painful—so painful sometimes that it can severely disrupt a person's eating.

Canker sores are found anywhere in the mouth: the inside of the cheeks, the lips, the sides of the tongue, the floor of the mouth, the gums, and the palate. They heal by themselves in about two weeks without leaving scars. Unfortunately, they tend to recur. Some people develop them every few weeks, others every few months, and some unlucky few are never without them.

Although no one knows what causes these painful mouth sores, many of the following triggering factors have been suspected:

- Poor dental hygiene.
- Foods such as chocolate, citrus fruits, spices, milk, cola drinks, and nuts, especially English walnuts.
- Allergies to drugs. Some common offenders are aspirin, antibiotics, sulfa drugs, and chemotherapeutic agents.
- Allergy to denture materials.
- Illness accompanied by fever.
- Menstruation
- Fatigue
- Emotional stress and tension.
- Injury caused by stiff toothbrushes or poorly fitting dentures.
- Viruses (similar to the viral infection responsible for cold sores).
- Bacteria
- Many patients have told me that shortly after they had given up smoking, they began to develop canker sores. And when they started to smoke again, the sores disappeared never to return. (However, I do not recommend smoking to alleviate or prevent canker sores!)

If you have recurrent canker sores the following general measures may prevent attacks:

- Keep your mouth clean.
- Avoid all kinds of nuts and any foods you suspect might be triggering factors,
- No chewing gum, mouthwashes, and menthol cigarettes.
- If you are using a fluoridated toothpaste (and who isn't?),

switch to a nonfluoridated brand (Peak or Viadent), or use salt or baking soda as a substitute.

- If they appear before your menstrual period, take an antihistamine daily, beginning a week or ten days before.

If none of these measures help, consult a dermatologist or dentist. Either one may be able to pinpoint the cause of your sores and suggest additional measures.

Theories on treating an existing attack of canker sores are almost as varied as the suspected causes. Among the many treatments that dermatologists and dentists recommend are dental ointments containing a "relative" of cortisone, painting the sores with silver nitrate solution, injecting a cortisone-like drug beneath the ulcers, and using lozenges of one kind or another.

There is, however, only one good, proven reliable method of relieving the pain due to canker sores: using mouthwashes or "compresses" that have tetracycline. Tetracycline is a prescription antibiotic and must be ordered by your doctor. This treatment involves emptying a 250-milligram capsule of tetracycline into one ounce of warm water and shaking it up very well. (Tetracycline powder cannot be dissolved in water but forms a suspension when shaken.) Swish this solution around in your mouth for five or ten minutes every two or three hours or soak wads of cotton in it and apply to the sores. Both methods should give prompt relief.

TREATING CANKER SORES

Other than the tetracycline "gargles" mentioned above, there is no good, reliable, over-the-counter preparation that works for everybody.

You can, however, try treating your canker sores with tea bags at home. The tannic acid in tea, for some unexplained reason, helps heal the sores.

Directions: Immerse a tea bag in tepid water, remove it, and squeeze out most of the water. Then apply the tea bag directly to the canker sore. You may be pleasantly surprised at the result.

For those who are plagued with recurrent canker sores, I recommend that you eat at least four tablespoonfuls of unflavored yogurt every day. If you do this daily, you may never have a canker sore again!

DIAPER RASH

Diaper rash, the bane of young mothers, the frustration of young fathers, and often the challenge of seasoned pediatricians, is a very common skin ailment. Beginning for the most part between the ages of two and four months, this itchy, burning, painful, nasty-looking rash can result in restlessness, irritability, and sleep interruption, and can persist for months or until your child outgrows diapers.

Also known as napkin or diaper dermatitis, diaper rash is an eruption on an infant's buttocks, genital and anal areas, lower abdomen, and upper thighs that manifests itself during the diaper-wearing stage. Although the problem is usually a minor one, it can, when ignored, lead to widespread infection by bacteria or fungi necessitating vigorous and prolonged treatment.

In its early and simple form, diaper rash is characterized by redness or chafing of the skin that is covered by the diaper. When left untreated, small pimples (called papules) and water blisters (called vesicles) develop. This can progress to oozing, sogginess in the skin folds and, in severe cases, open sores. The sharp, pungent odor of ammonia usually accompanies this rash.

It is a truism to say that the villain in all cases of diaper rash is, sad to day, the diaper. Babies do not, and cannot, develop diaper rash if they do not wear diapers! In our society, however, it is de rigueur for our infants to sport diapers: cloth, synthetic, treated, odor-preventing, and a host of other types and styles. Greek babies do not develop diaper rash because they are regularly cleansed by their mothers who cradle them in their left arm while the right arm washes away the urine and soilings under a stream of warm tap water.

Other causes of diaper rash include rubber or plastic pants which constrict and prevent the skin that is covered by the diaper from "breathing." This can be further aggravated by the rough edges of these pants as well as by tightly-pinned diapers.

Frequent loose stools with their noxious intestinal enzymes can irritate the delicate diaper area, especially when these stools have not been completely removed by cleaning. Other causes of irritation include harsh soaps for cleaning the skin; strong detergents, antiseptic rinses, and perfumed fabric softeners; and assorted baby oils, salves, ointments, and other chemical irritants.

High heat and humidity also contribute to diaper rash as they cause the skin and skin folds to become water-logged. This creates an inflammation around the sweat pores and prevents the normal flow of perspiration, thus lowering the resistance of the skin to infection. The normal, usually "friendly" and harmless germs, such as bacteria and fungi, then begin to thrive and set up housekeeping in these trapped fluids and become "unfriendly" and harmful.

Although the situation often seem dismal, there are some positive steps you can take to prevent and treat diaper rash. Here are a few suggestions for prevention:

- Use soft, cotton diapers.
- Change diapers as soon as they are soiled *and* at regular intervals. Newborns urinate more than twenty times a day, and one-year olds average six or seven times a day. Therefore, be on the alert and learn to anticipate.
- Use plastic and rubber pants only sparingly and for short periods of time, such as for party occasions. Never use them at night.
- Following each diaper change, clean the diaper area thoroughly but gently with a mild cleanser, such as Cetaphil Lotion, to remove all bacterial and fecal contamination. Pay careful attention to the skin folds. These folds should be washed gently and then rinsed thoroughly to make certain that all the cleanser is completely removed.
- Dry the skin and the skin folds thoroughly.
- Use a medicated cornstarch-based powder two or three times daily to keep the affected areas dry.
- Wash diapers in mild soap or detergent. Make sure they are carefully and painstakingly rinsed.
- Don't use the perfumed fabric softener pads that are placed in clothes dryers.
- Dress your child in clothing that is porous enough to allow good air circulation.
- Keep air in the child's room cool and dry.
- Encourage early training in regular toilet habits.

If your child is already suffering from diaper rash, the following steps can help clear it up and forestall further irritation, inflammation, and infection.

- Stop all previous medication.
- Discontinue plastic and rubber pants.
- Never use soap when the skin is inflamed.
- Apply wet dressings, compresses, or 15-minute baths using Burow's Solution (two Bluboro packets dissolved in one quart of warm water) every three or four hours to soothe and cool the inflamed areas.
- Allow the affected areas to "breathe." Air is a marvelous healing agent! I strongly recommend that you permit infants and children with diaper rash to lie about and run around naked for several hours a day! Remember: there cannot be a diaper rash without diapers.

During the acute stage of diaper rash, I urge that you discontinue *all* diapers during the day. Use a double layer of soft, cotton diapers, very loosely pinned, at night. Never use plastic or rubber pants at any time.

When the inflammation, oozing, and sogginess have begun to clear and dry up, use a soothing and protective preparation, such as zinc oxide paste, at night. Finally, when the affected areas have adequately healed and the child is more comfortable, you may use soft cotton diapers again.

Be especially careful and conscientious, change the sheets as often as necessary, wash the soiled areas gently but thoroughly, and reapply the zinc oxide paste after each soiling.

TREATING DIAPER RASH
For the weeping and oozing of acute diaper rash, apply soothing wet dressings of the following to help relieve the inflammation and make the child more comfortable:

Bluboro Powder Packets (Herbert)

Directions: Dissolve the contents of one packet in a pint (16 ounces) of warm water and apply as open wet dressings for fifteen to twenty minutes every two or three hours. (See page 217 for directions for applying wet dressings.)

After the acute inflammation has subsided with the wet dressings, apply the following:

Zinc Oxide Paste

Directions: Apply at night to the affected areas.

DIMPLE WARTS

Dimple warts are benign (friendly) skin tumors caused by a virus, the largest of all true viruses known to cause human disease. The scientific name for these growths is molluscum contagiosum.

These warts occur most frequently in children and young adults. They do not itch, hurt, or burn, but they are highly contagious. They can spread indirectly (through towels, washcloths, and similar items) or directly from person to person. Epidemics of these viral tumors are common among children and adolescents in schools, orphanages, and other institutions. In sexually active people it is considered a sexually transmitted disease.

It usually takes about six weeks from the time of contact or exposure to the virus until the disease appears. The virus enters the skin through small injuries (scratches, insect bites, or puncture wounds). The tumors usually begin as pinhead-sized elevations which gradually enlarge to the size of a small pea. They may persist for years but usually stop growing once they reach this size.

The elevations, known as nodules, are smooth, round, dome-shaped, and either waxy or pearly in appearance. Older molluscums usually develop a dimple resembling a bellybutton (hence the name: dimple wart). The lesions are often confined to the abdomen, thighs, pubic area, and genitals, but can occur on any portion of the skin surface. Non-sexual transmission of the condition is often seen in wrestlers.

When squeezed, dimple warts discharge a milky-white, curd-like substance. Left untreated, they usually disappear by themselves after months or years without leaving scars. Since they are contagious, however, there are some measures you should take.

Avoid touching the people you know have the virus, and practice good hygiene (keep clean!). A dermatologist can eradicate them quickly and almost painlessly by any of a variety of methods. One popular technique is to freeze them off with liquid nitrogen. They also can be burned off (cauterized) under local anesthesia, scraped off with a small curette (actually a "round knife"), or destroyed with various chemicals. All of these procedures are safe and effective.

TREATING DIMPLE WARTS

Since dimple warts are viral tumors, it is often difficult to get rid of them with anything except surgical or freezing techniques used by a dermatologist. The following preparation, however, may help destroy an "early" wart:

Wart Medicine (Dr. Scholl's)

Directions: Apply once daily—*very carefully*—to the top of each dimple wart. Stop if irritation occurs.

If, after a couple of weeks, the warts show no sign of budging or if new lesions have appeared, see your dermatologist.

FROSTBITE

Frostbite—the sharp, painful sensations that result from the freezing and thawing of the skin. It is a severe cold injury that, in many ways, resembles the burn you get when you touch something hot. Press an ice cube on your cheeks for a few seconds. Burns, doesn't it? If you were to leave it there for a few minutes, you would develop a painful blister.

Whether exposure to cold will result in frostbite depends on many factors, including the temperature, the wind-chill factor, how long you're exposed, and what you're wearing. People's tolerance to cold varies as well. There are several conditions that reduce one's tolerance: poor circulation, poor general health, poor nutrition, fatigue, injury, immobility of an extremity, and contact with metals.

The areas of the body most vulnerable to the effects of frostbite are the feet and toes, the tip of the nose, the rims and lobes of the ears, and the tips of the fingers.

How do you recognize frostbite? In its mildest form, known as frost nip, the skin suddenly turns pale due to the constriction of blood vessels. This is the body's method of conserving heat by diverting the blood to the vital internal organs. This skin pallor is accompanied by tingling. Burning and pain follow, and the skin becomes whitish or slightly yellow.

If the freezing continues, it affects the deeper tissues. The pain disappears and areas affected become numb (Disappearance of pain is a warning sign of imminent danger!). The affected skin then becomes waxy white. Severe and lengthy exposure to cold can injure deeper tissues, such as muscles, tendons, nerves, and bones.

Children who suffer severe cases of frostbitten fingers often end up with small hands as adults.

If you develop frostbite, see your doctor at once. Do not treat it with ice, ice-water, or snow. This "cold" treatment can actually kill the tissue. And do not move any skin that is frozen: movement will result in severe damage. Also, don't smoke or drink alcohol.

The best method to treat frostbite—the one that your doctor will probably recommend—is to restore the normal temperature of the skin by *rapidly* rewarming the frostbitten area. Immerse the affected part in a water bath at a temperature of 104° to 110° F (40° to 44° C). Better yet, use a whirlpool bath. Make sure the temperature doesn't exceed 110° F. Because your skin doesn't have any sensation, you could produce a burn at higher temperatures. Do not use local, dry heat. And do not move the frozen skin. This treatment may produce more pain, more redness and swelling, and bigger blisters than gradual rewarming, but it promotes faster healing, reduces tissue loss, and prevents complications, such as infection, ulceration, gangrene, and even loss of a limb.

During the thawing process, blisters will develop. These blisters may persist for weeks, and the newly formed skin may be tender for months. In most cases of mild to moderate frostbite, complete healing will usually take place in a week or two.

To guard against frostbite, dress normally and protect those parts that are most susceptible to cold. When the temperature falls and the wind is howling, causing the chill factor to drop to arctic levels, protect those delicate sensitive areas: the fingertips with warm gloves or mittens; the ears with muffs or flaps; and the nose with a ski mask. The feet should be enclosed in thick, loose-fitting, lined boots that can accommodate thick socks. Protect the rest of the body with thermal underwear, long-johns, turtle neck sweaters, scarves, and fur-lined coats. The ideal fabric for outdoors wear is one that traps a lot of air. Loosely woven bulky wool or acrylic, Thinsulate, Hollowfil, and PolarGuard all fill this guideline.

Keep up your general health and avoid fatigue.

TREATING FROSTBITE

The recommended procedure for treating frostbite is to soak the affected part in a water bath at a temperature of 104° to 110° F (40° to 44° C).

For the blisters that may develop during the thawing process, apply wet compresses for 15 to 20 minutes every 2 or 3 hours with the following antiseptic solution:

Bluboro Powder (Herbert)

Directions for use are on the container. The temperature of the solution should be the same as above.

When the blisters have begun to dry up, you may discontinue the compresses.

FUNGOUS INFECTIONS OF THE SKIN

ATHLETE'S FOOT

Athlete's foot does attack the feet, but it's not limited to athletes. It's also known as ringworm, but it's not a worm. Having disposed of two popular misconceptions about an ailment that gets a toehold on so many of us, let's get down to the facts.

Athlete's foot is a nasty infection caused by a fungus. It occurs mostly among teenage and adult males. It is fairly easy to treat, but it can be stubborn, too. Although the majority of fungous infections of the skin are not life-threatening, the effects on the quality of life can be significant.

Fungous diseases, or disease caused by a fungus, are very common skin disorders. Fungi are living germs, actually miniature plants, which grow and multiply on the skin, in the hair, and in the nails of almost all living creatures.

(All fungi, by the way, are not harmful; many are beneficial and play a role in producing beer, cheese, and antibiotics such as penicillin. Other fungi, however, cause rust, mildew, and ringworm infections.)

Why certain people develop fungous infections and others do not are questions that have not yet been resolved. Why females have a lower incidence is also unknown. Perhaps women are cleaner, sweat less, wash more often, and wear looser footgear. Maybe their hormones have antifungal properties. We really don't know. There is speculation that some people are immune to certain types of infections, and ringworm may be one of these.

Ringworm of the feet does not occur in primitive races accustomed to going barefoot, and it almost never appears in children under the age of twelve. Thus, if your child has a rash on his or her feet, it probably is *not* a fungous infection.

It is possible to be a host of the fungus of athlete's foot without any infection or other symptoms. It is only when you lower the natural resistance of the skin that the fungi thrive, proliferate, invade the outer layers of the skin, and set up housekeeping. This lowered resistance may be the result of excessive moisture and sweating (particularly in the summertime, due to sweaty socks and not drying your feet after swimming and bathing), inadequate ventilation of the feet (tight shoes and socks), uncleanliness, or friction.

Athlete's foot affects people in different ways. For some it is characterized by peeling, cracking, and scaling of the skin between the toes (particularly between the last two toes). Other people experience redness, scaling, and blisters along the sides and soles of the feet. Occasionally there is intense itching. Still other people develop a dry, reddish, non-itchy, scaly eruption, covering the entire sole. This common infection is referred to as the moccasin, or sandal, type of athlete's foot.

By the way, every rash on the feet is not necessarily athlete's foot: it may be an allergy from shoes or dyes, it may be psoriasis, or any of a number of conditions that frequently attack the feet and toes.

If you have a persistent rash on your feet, consult your physician. Over-the-counter medications may only aggravate conditions that have been misdiagnosed as athlete's foot. And, if left untreated, athlete's foot can lead to infection by other organisms—bacteria. This may require antibiotic therapy, continuous wet dressings, and complete bed rest. Only your doctor can diagnosis athlete's foot with any certainty.

How do you treat athlete's foot? No problem.

In the simple, uncomplicated cases, I recommend applying antifungal creams or gels to the affected areas twice daily. This will usually cure the condition in a matter of weeks. If there is weeping, oozing, and blisters, and if the toewebs are wet and soggy, you should soak your feet twice a day in Burow's Solution (see below) before applying the antifungal medication.

If your athlete's foot is stubborn and extensive, or if it has settled in and affected your toenails, or if you have an allergic spread on your fingers and hands in the form of itchy water blisters, your doctor will probably prescribe some newer topical creams and lotions (Loprox, Nizoral, Naftin), and, perhaps, oral antifungal medications.

How can you prevent athlete's foot?

- Wash your feet at least once daily.
- Keep them meticulously dry at all times—use a blow dryer if necessary.

- Wear only one hundred percent cotton socks and change them daily. Never wear socks that contain any synthetic materials; these are occlusive and cause sweating.
- Avoid tight or snug footwear in hot, humid weather (perforated shoes or sandals are best).
- Dust an antifungal powder into your shoes in the summertime.

If you follow all the suggestions mentioned above, you will never be tripped up by athlete's foot.

TREATING ATHLETE'S FOOT

In the acute stage, when your toewebs and toes are red, oozing, and blistered, do not apply any surface medication. The only helpful therapy at this stage is to soak your feet in antiseptic solutions every four or six hours. See pages 218 for the proper method to soak the feet. The following compress should be used:

Bluboro Powder (Herbert)

Directions: Dissolve contents of one packet in a pint (16 ounces) of warm water as soaks as directed above.

During the soaking process, keep your toewebs separated by thin strips of linen or cotton material, such as old washed sheets or shirts or handkerchiefs. Never use cotton balls or batting, as their wood fiber content can be irritating.

CREAM, GEL

After the soaking, or when the lesions have begun to dry up, apply any of the following to the affected areas:

Tinactin Cream (Schering)

Micatin Antifungal Cream (Ortho)

Antinea Antifungal Cream (American Dermal)

POWDER

Dust the following powder on your feet and between your toes twice daily:

Zeasorb AF Powder (Stiefel)

While treating athlete's foot, it is important to keep your toes separated. Purchase lamb's wool from your drugstore, and use it day and night.

JOCK ITCH

Jock itch is one of those conditions, like hemorrhoids, that few people talk about in public. But there are a lot of people who suffer from it in private.

Jock itch is a common infection of the groin area in young men which often occurs in association with athlete's foot. While the term "jock itch" is the popular expression that describes any rash in the groin area, it usually indicates a superficial fungous (ringworm) infection caused by the same organisms—miniature plants called fungi—that can give you athlete's foot.

Jock itch occurs more frequently in summertime. It commonly affects plump people and people who are physically active. The tiny fungi that cause jock itch often live harmlessly on the skin, but when exposed to the right conditions—hot, humid, and damp places such as locker rooms, shower stalls, and swimming pools— they begin to thrive, multiply, and become harmful.

The groin area is more susceptible to skin irritation and infection than other parts of the body for several reasons. Groins are wet, warm, and dark. The skin is thin and delicate, and subject to friction, particularly if you do a lot of strenuous activity or if you have some extra folds of fat to chafe against your clothing. In addition, jockey shorts, tight pants, jock straps, and wet bathing suits not only make you sweat more, but they prevent evaporation, making the groin area ideally suited for the growth and proliferation of these infectious organisms.

Jock itch usually begins as a small, reddish, scaly rash in the groin area which gradually enlarges to form a patch with a sharply-defined border. If left untreated, the rash may spread to involve the upper inner thighs, the scrotum, the buttocks, and the pubic and anal areas. The skin becomes raw and soggy due to moisture and friction. Itching is the most common symptom, but there also may be some burning and pain.

How can you prevent jock itch? And if you have it already, how can you treat it?

Here are some general measures to prevent jock itch:

- Personal cleanliness (soap and water daily) is a must. Don't, however, scrub too hard. This may injure the upper layers of the skin and, as a result, compromise the body's natural defense mechanism which prevents invasion by harmful germs.
- After washing, rinse, and dry thoroughly. A blow dryer can often help.
- Reduce perspiration.

- Help the sweat evaporate by proper ventilation. Wear loose-fitting, cotton, underwear and loose pants. Air is a deterrent to the growth of these fungi.
- Change your underwear at least daily; underwear is a good breeding place for ringworm germs.
- Put your socks on before your undershorts. This will prevent dragging some of the fungi from your feet up to your groin.
- Wash your hands after touching your feet and toes.
- Don't wear anyone else's underwear.
- Treat any athlete's foot you may have developed.

TREATING JOCK ITCH

In the acute stage of jock itch, when there's redness, burning, and pain, do not apply any creams or powders to the affected areas. The only treatment that will alleviate this phase is to soak the areas in a tub of warm water. This will soothe the burning and itching and help dry up wet, weeping areas.

After the baths, apply the following twice daily:

Tinactin Cream (Schering)

When the rash is nearly healed, dust an antifungal powder—*Zeasorb AF Powder* (Stiefel)—in the groin areas twice daily to prevent a recurrence of the jock itch.

Also, it's important to treat any athlete's foot you may have. No athlete's foot, no jock itch.

TINEA VERSICOLOR

Tinea versicolor is a friendly, minor fungous infection of the skin. Friendly means that it is relatively harmless; minor means that it is only mildly contagious (through direct contact and clothing) and, for the most part, is easy to cure. While it lasts, however, it can be itchy and, when widespread, may be embarrassing cosmetically.

Like most fungous infections, tinea versicolor thrives in hot, humid environments. During the summer months, people often complain about itching and scaling; in winter, many of the symptoms disappear. Some people are more predisposed to this condition than others, and adolescents and young adults seem to be most susceptible.

The name tinea versicolor means "superficial fungous infection characterized by a change of color." To establish a diagnosis of this condition, a physician will scrape some of the scales off one of the patches and search for the responsible fungus. Under the microscope, the fungus looks like a dish of spaghetti and meatballs—small spherical spores and rod-like filaments. (Dermatologists refer to it as the "spaghetti-and-meatball" fungus.)

To the eye, tinea versicolor appears as fine, round, scaly patches that usually are tan or fawn-colored. These patches are most common over the chest, back, and shoulders. Acting as a sunscreen, they block out the sun's rays. In white people this results in depigmented areas of the skin that are lighter than the surrounding, tanned skin in summer and darker than the surrounding, untanned skin in winter. In black people these depigmented patches can be various colors: tan, brown, gray, yellow, or even pink.

Tinea versicolor is easy to treat and leaves no scars. Since the condition has a tendency to recur, however, particularly in hot, humid weather, you may have to continue treatment over a long period of time. If left untreated, the condition may persist indefinitely.

Treatment usually consists of washing the affected areas with a prescription-type shampoo containing selenium sulfide (Selsun). Over-the-counter shampoos, such as Selsun Blue, DHS Zinc Shampoo, or ZNP Bar also can do a pretty good job. Washing the affected areas for a full five minutes once daily for period of two weeks will usually eliminate most of the active fungus. Monthly washings thereafter should prevent the condition from recurring. I also recommend thoroughly shampooing the scalp at least once weekly with the same shampoo, since the fungus often sets up housekeeping in the back of the scalp. You may use other shampoos in between. Once you have begun treatment, it is important to wear freshly laundered or dry-cleaned clothing to prevent reinfection.

A relatively new oral medication, ketoconazole, is being used by many dermatologists to treat tinea versicolor. Only two tablets are required to destroy the fungus, but there are certain adverse side effects to this medication.

Even after you have destroyed the fungus, the patches may require repeated sun exposure to change back to their normal color. This may take months, so be patient!

TREATING TINEA VERSICOLOR
Wash the affected areas thoroughly for five minutes daily for a period of two weeks. Repeat these washings monthly for at least a year. Use any of the following "washes":
ZNP Bar (Stiefel)

DHS Zinc Shampoo (Person & Covey)
Selsun Blue (Abbott)

Shampoo your scalp at least once weekly with the same "wash."

ICHTHYOSIS

Ichthyosis, or "fishskin disease," is a relatively uncommon, hereditary condition. There are four distinct types of these coarse, rough, and scaly skin disorders all of which are characterized by an increase in the thickness of the upper layers of the skin.

Brought about by abnormalities in either protein or fat metabolism, these diseases are a result of either an excessive production of skin cells, or as a consequence of increased "stickiness" of the uppermost layer of the skin, the horny layer, which occasions an impairment in the normal shedding process.

(The upper layer of the skin, the epidermis, is constantly regenerating itself: all its cells turn themselves over about every 28 days. Dead cells slough off as new ones push up in a perpetual and lifelong process of cell division. It takes about two weeks for the newborn cells to make their way to the outermost layer of the epidermis, where they remain, as dead and dying cells, for another two weeks until they are cast off. See the chapter on Dandruff.)

The two most prevalent types of ichthyosis are ichthyosis vulgaris and X-linked ichthyosis. In both types, the normal shedding process is retarded.

The most common, or "vulgar," type of ichthyosis, known appropriately as ichthyosis vulgaris, develops after the first three months of life and affects one in every three hundred people. It is inherited, may affect several members of a family, and is characterized by fine, white, branny scaling which appears most prominently over the trunk and outside surfaces of the arms and legs. The inside of the elbow and knee areas, the flexures, are not involved, but the palms and soles are often thickened. There is no itching or burning or other subjective symptoms; the chief complaints of this fishlike, scaly disorder are cosmetic in nature.

Ichthyosis vulgaris gets better with age and with warm, moist surroundings, and is often associated with some form of allergy—eczema, hay fever, or asthma—and with dry skin of the palms and heels which is intensified in cold, dry weather.

The second most common type of inherited scaly skin is called

X-linked ichthyosis. This more severe variety affects about one in 6,000 males and is transmitted to sons by unaffected mothers. As in ichthyosis vulgaris, this variant results from retarded shedding of the uppermost layers of the skin.

Characterized by early onset, from birth until about one year, and generalized involvement, this condition displays large, coarse, adherent, "stuck-on" scales over the neck, trunk, buttocks, and outer portions of the extremities. When the neck is affected, it invariably has an unwashed appearance. X-linked ichthyosis becomes increasingly severe with the passage of time.

While there is no cure for ichthyosis, various therapies can greatly improve the appearance of the skin and relieve the excessive dryness and scaling. If the person lives in a warm, humid environment, little treatment is required for either type of ichthyosis just described. Keeping the relative humidity levels above 60 percent is vital.

TREATING ICHTHYOSIS

The topical application of soothing, lotions, creams, and ointments immediately following comforting oil baths is all that is necessary in the milder cases. Deodorant and other harsh soaps are poorly tolerated.

SOAPS
Try any of the following soaps:
Alpha Keri Moisturizing Bar (Westwood)
Basis Soap (Beiersdorf)
Oilatum Soap (Stiefel)

BATH OILS
Alpha Keri Bath Oil (Westwood)
Nutraderm Bath Oil (Owen)
Hermal Bath Oil (Hermal)
Directions for use on the labels.

EMOLLIENT CREAMS AND LOTIONS
Moisturel Cream and Lotion (Westwood)
NutraPlus Cream and Lotion (Owen)
Epilyt Lotion (Stiefel)
Directions: Apply to affected areas as often as needed.

A breakthrough in the treatment of ichthyosis has recently come about with the use of topical preparations containing lactic acid and its derivatives. The most notable of these is Lac-Hydrin Lotion, a prescription medication that when applied locally as directed is exceptionally effective in reducing the excessive scaling that is typical of the ichthyoses.

Vitamin A, when taken in moderately large doses under the supervision of a dermatologist, often helps.

For further information about ichthyosis, write to:

Foundation for Ichthyosis & Related Skin Types, Inc.
3640 Grand Avenue, Suite 2
Oakland, California 94610
Valerie Lutters, Acting Executive Director
415/763-9839

LICHEN PLANUS

Lichen planus is a relatively common, harmless, noncontagious, itchy rash that involves the skin and mucous membranes. Occurring most commonly in the middle years, it is characterized by reddish or violet-colored, firm, shiny, flat-topped, diamond-shaped "bumps," called papules.

The rash of lichen planus usually is symmetrical in appearance and most often involves the inner surfaces of the wrists and forearms, the ankles, and the lower portion of the back. No area of the skin surface, however, is immune from this condition.

In the mouth, lichen planus can appear as a whitish or bluish-white, lacy-like pattern on the inner surface of the cheeks, or as whitish patches over the sides of the tongue. In rarer forms of this disorder, blisters or thickened warty areas may appear. In addition, one out of ten people with lichen planus have some type of nail changes, such as grooves, lines, distortion, or shedding of the nails.

The most characteristic symptom of lichen planus is itching. If there are only a few patches of the condition, the itching is usually mild. In the generalized form of the disease, however, the itching may become intense, causing loss of sleep, exhaustion, and despair.

The cause of lichen planus is unknown. It may be that it is not a disease at all, rather a symptom resulting from irritation, inflammation, or infection somewhere in the body.

Lichen planus can occur in people taking various drugs: high-blood pressure pills, antibiotics, and certain medications used to treat tuberculosis, malaria, and arthritis. The condition can also develop in workers in the photographic chemical industry following exposure to a type of color film developer. Many cases of resistant lichen planus occur in association with long-standing, untreated fungous infections of the feet (athlete's foot). Since the onset of lichen planus occasionally coincides with some major emotional upset, it is often thought to be triggered by prolonged worry, anxiety, fatigue, shock, or other stressful situation.

Lichen planus can last for years, but as a rule, the greater the involvement, the shorter the course. Generalized and extensive eruptions last anywhere from two months to two years. Localized eruptions, on the other hand, have a tendency to remain considerably longer. Unfortunately, recurrences are common, so one is never sure that the condition has disappeared permanently.

While fairly common, lichen planus is not a condition that is easily recognized and diagnosed by the person who is afflicted— or by relatives, friends, or the friendly pharmacist. Only a physician, specifically a dermatologist, can make an accurate diagnosis, and while there is no specific therapy for lichen planus, your physician will know how best to treat the rash and the itching that accompany it.

Available treatments include various cortisone-like creams applied locally, certain antihistamine tranquilizers taken orally, and cortisone-like injections into the patches of lichen planus. None of these, however, has shown more than limited success.

If you have a rash that has been diagnosed by your physician as lichen planus, be content to know that it is not contagious, infectious, serious, or malignant. Get as much rest as possible and avoid worry, tension, and fatigue. Maintain your general health and correct any hidden, internal infection you may have, such as abscessed teeth or infected gums.

TREATMENT OF LICHEN PLANUS

As discussed above, itching is probably the most obvious symptom of lichen planus. It is also the most difficult symptom to control.

The localized patches are best managed with creams, ointments, and gels. Either of the following preparations may provide some symptomatic relief:

Hytone Cream 0.5% (Dermik) or
Cort-Aid Ointment (Upjohn)
Directions for use are on the packages.

For the extensive or generalized variety of lichen planus, soothing baths, once daily, are often palliative. Use either
Nutraderm Bath Oil (Owen) or
Balnetar (Westwood)
Directions for each on the labels.
Also try either of the following lotions for the extensive cases, two or three times daily:
Schamberg's Lotion (C&M Pharmacal) or
Sarna Lotion (Stiefel)
For the itching that invariably accompanies the rash of lichen planus, take either of the following antihistamines every four hours when necessary:
Chlor-Trimeton Tablets [4 mg] (Schering) or
Dimetane Tablets [4 mg] (Robins)
Directions and cautions on the labels.
For persistent, unmanageable itching, and when none of the above medications offers any relief, it is important to see your dermatologist.

LUPUS
ERYTHEMATOSUS

"The wolf, I'm afraid, is inside tearing up the place. I've
been in the hospital 50 days already this year."
Flannery O'Connor (a few days before succumbing to her
progressive and inexorable fatal illness).

Lupus erythematosus is one of those curious diseases that can masquerade as any of a dozen other medical maladies. Its variety of symptoms include, fever, chills, headache, weakness, fatigue, hair loss, joint pains, chest pain, epileptic seizures, personality changes, and skin rashes. Any or all of these symptoms may be part of this complicated disease we commonly call LE.
What exactly is LE? It is a chronic inflammation of connective tissue—the so-called body "glue"—that binds our cells together. As such, it is considered a connective tissue, or collagen, disease and is often classified in the rheumatic group of diseases along with rheumatic fever and rheumatoid arthritis. Every part of our bodies—all our organs, our muscles, blood, joints, skin—has this connective tissue, and thus, may be affected by LE.
No one really knows what causes LE. This puzzling condition,

which affects over 500,000 people in the United States, is most likely due to an "autoimmune process"—a technical way of saying that the body, due to some unexplained allergy, produces certain abnormal substances called autoantibodies that attack and destroy its own tissues. Normally, when foreign substances (antigens), such as disease-producing germs or allergens, attack your body, it responds by producing antibodies to fight off these harmful invaders. In people with LE, this normal defense mechanism breaks down. And instead of attacking the antigens, the antibodies attack the body's own tissues. A most difficult concept to comprehend.

It is important to know there are two types of LE. One is the benign or "friendly" type, called the discoid variety of LE. Triggered by some external factor such as sunlight or injury, it shows up as red, scaly patches symmetrically distributed over the sun-exposed areas of the body—the cheeks, nose, ears, scalp, the backs of the hands, and occasionally the "V" of the neck. The patches of LE, thought to resemble (on the face) the teeth marks of a wolf—hence the word lupus—can also affect the beard and scalp, usually resulting in permanent hair loss.

These patches grow larger over a period of months or years, forming disc-shaped (hence, discoid) patches. They slowly lose their reddish color, and become white and depressed. This depression—essentially a scar, is the end result of a typical discoid lesion.

Discoid LE affects all races, is more common in young adults, and occurs twice as often in women as in men. If you have discoid LE, it's important to see a dermatologist. While the condition itself is relatively harmless, these "discs" may be harbingers of some underlying condition that can flare up into systemic lupus erythematosus (SLE).

SLE is a serious variety of LE that can affect and damage any or all of the body's organs or systems: kidneys, liver, heart, lungs, bone marrow, and joints. Fortunately, only about one in ten people with discoid LE ever progress to the systemic or internal type of the disease.

One of the triggering mechanisms that may convert the "friendly" condition into the more serious, "unfriendly" variety is sun exposure. People with LE, therefore, must strictly avoid the beaches, sunbathing in general, and tropical cruises.

Other factors that can turn the "benign" form of the disease into the more serious type, are stress, injury, fatigue, overwork, certain medications (such as those used for high blood pressure, heart disease, and epilepsy), antibiotics and birth control pills, various types of tranquilizers, and after exposure in tanning salons.

Treatment for LE will depend on your age and the nature and severity of your symptoms. Your dermatologist may prescribe cortisone-like creams and ointments to reduce the redness and relieve the inflammation in the affected patches. In rare cases, where the lesions are progressive, widespread, or disfiguring, your doctor may prescribe drugs called antimalarials to prevent further spread.

For further information regarding LE, write to:

National Lupus Erythematosus Foundation
5430 Van Nuys Boulevard, Suite #206
Van Nuys, California 91401
818/885-8787
Marlene Rothstein, Director

TREATING LUPUS ERYTHEMATOSUS

The treatment for LE is up to your physician. However, to prevent aggravating the condition, always use a "high-powered" sunscreen before sun exposure. Use either of the following:

PreSun 39 (Westwood)
Solbar 15 Plus (Person & Covey)

For any itching that is associated with LE patches, use the following cream three or four times daily:

Hytone Cream 0.5% (Dermik)

Cosmetic coverups, such as Covermark or Dermablend, can be used to hide any disfiguring scars.

PRICKLY HEAT

Prickly heat is a common disorder of the sweat apparatus. It arises when the free flow of sweat to the surface of the skin is obstructed. The medical term for this condition is miliaria.

Sweat is produced by the more than 2 million sweat glands in the skin. Under normal conditions, it flows out smoothly and uninterruptedly to the skin surface through tiny sweat ducts. If the sweat is heavy and prolonged, it can clog the ducts and become trapped. This trapped sweat, unable to reach the skin surface,

breaks through the walls of the ducts. The result is an inflammation of the skin known as prickly heat, or heat rash.

While prickly heat can materialize at any age, there is a
tendency for it to occur more commonly in infants for two reasons:
the relatively small size of the sweat ducts encourages closing of
the pores thereby favoring sweat retention, and parent's instinc-
tive overprotection of the infant from the cold contributes to the
warmth and humidity in which heat rash flourishes.

Prickly heat often appears suddenly and takes the form of
numerous, tiny, reddish pimples and water blisters scattered in the
creases of the neck, under the chin, in the armpits, and on the
chest, back, abdomen, and buttocks. Recurrent crops may continue indefinitely and can cause restlessness and irritability, as
well as burning and prickling sensations.

Prickly heat can result from any condition that encourages
profuse and prolonged sweating along with inadequate evaporation of the sweat. The offender can be an excessively hot and humid
climate or a fever. Indeed, persistent and extensive cases of heat
rash are most common in tropical climes. Aggravated by obesity
and tightly-fitting garments, prickly heat usually clears up on its
own, and only rarely do complications, such as secondary bacterial
and fungal infections, materialize. While it lasts, however, it can
be very distressing, particularly for young children.

There are, fortunately, some simple and effective methods to
prevent and treat prickly heat. The primary concern is to keep the
skin cool and dry. This is easy: keep the *air* cool and dry. Other
helpful suggestions include the following:

- Use an air-conditioner or fan to reduce the temperature and
  humidity.
- Maintain adequate room ventilation to help the evaporation
  of sweat.
- Dress your child in loose-fitting, lightweight cotton clothing
  and limit physical activity in hot, humid weather.

If prickly heat has already taken place, try the following
treatment:

- Apply soothing and drying lotions, such as plain calamine
  lotion.
- Use a cornstarch-based dusting powder.

- If possible, allow the afflicted child to lie about the house naked.
- Wash with a cleanser, such as Cetaphil Lotion, and never use greases or ointments which will further clog the sweat ducts.
- During the acute phase of prickly heat, take lukewarm baths, preferably with Linit Starch or Aveeno Bath Regular Formula.

Of course, the main answer to prickly heat is to stay cool!

TREATING PRICKLY HEAT
BATHS
Aveeno Bath Regular Formula (Rydelle) or
Linit Starch
Directions: See directions on the labels.

CLEANSING AGENTS
Cetaphil Lotion (Owen/Galderma) or
Lowila Cake (Westwood)

POWDER
Diaparene Baby Powder (Glenbrook)

LOTION
Calamine Lotion
Directions: Apply 2 or 3 times daily and after the bath.

RECTAL ITCH

One bliss for which
There is no match
Is when you itch
To up and scratch.

Ogden Nash's little ditty doesn't include the socially unmentionable, embarrassing itch that torments the anal area, often incorrectly referred to as the rectal area. Known technically as pruritus ani (itching of the anal region), this stubborn condition can cause sleepless nights, loss of work time, and severe emotional distress.

The single, most common cause of anal itch is poor anal hygiene. In most parts of Europe and in many Eastern countries this ailment is almost nonexistent. There many people do not use toilet tissue—they *wash* the area. (The bidet is a much more distinctive sign of civilization than we Americans would like to think!)

Other causes of anal itch include the following:

- Hemorrhoids (piles) and other rectal disease, such as fissures, fistulas, or discharge after rectal surgery.
- Chronic diarrhea.
- Fungous and yeast infections in the area—often associated with taking antibiotics over long periods.
- Pinworms and other parasitic infestations, such as lice (crabs) and mites (scabies).
- Psoriasis, seborrheic dermatitis, eczema.
- Warts in the anal area.
- Diabetes.
- Certain foods, such as coffee, spicy foods, chocolate, raw fruits and vegetables, and alcoholic beverages.
- Tight clothing, particularly the non-cotton varieties.
- Irritants that come into contact with the anal area, such as anesthetic ointments and suppositories used for piles; colored, perfumed, and coarse toilet paper; soaps (especially the colored and scented varieties); deodorants; feminine hygiene sprays; bath salts; and—believe it or not—even nail polish has been implicated.
- Psychogenic causes. Anal itching occurs twice as often in men in their 40s and 50s than in women of the same age. Physicians believe this to be a result of certain stress situations (monetary for the most part) that develop in middle-aged men.

And then there are those cases where one cannot determine the cause—where painstaking study has failed to reveal any causative factor. This is by far the most common situation, and, as a result, the most resistant to treatment.

If you have prolonged, continuous, intolerable anal itching, see a dermatologist. For temporary relief, here are a few things you can do:

- Never use dry toilet paper. Instead, use cotton soaked in warm water or use an anal cleaner such as Balneol. And never wipe or rub! Blotting or patting is enough. And make sure the area is kept scrupulously dry.

- Never use soap while you have "the itch."
- Avoid irritating substances, such as bath salts, deodorants, sprays, and perfumes. And do not dry your clothes with those perfumed fabric softeners.
- Avoid tight underwear, pajamas, and pants. Wear only loose, cotton clothes on your bottom half.
- If you suspect that diet may be responsible for your itch, cut our spicy foods, chocolate, coffee, alcohol, popcorn, and raw fruit and vegetables.
- Avoid antibiotics, laxatives, and mineral oil.
- Don't apply any over-the-counter salves and suppositories to the anal area, especially those containing benzocaine and other -caine derivatives. These may only aggravate your malady.
- If you suspect that emotional stress and tension are the cause, simmer down, stay cool, and relax.

For the severe, acute anal itch, your dermatologist will probably prescribe sitz baths in hot water, a special prescription cream or ointment, and perhaps an anti-itch pill to break that itch-scratch reflex.

How can you prevent anal itching? No problem. Keep the area scrupulously clean at all times and wash with a mild soap and water at least once daily (particularly after a bowel movement). Dry the area with soft, white toilet tissue. (Rabelais wrote that wiping the anal skin with the neck of a plump, downy, warm goose was unquestionably "the most lordly, excellent, and expedient technique ever seen.") Soft toilet paper is considerably easier to use, much cheaper, and probably works as well!

If you follow the cleansing and drying method just described, you may never again have to "up and scratch."

TREATING RECTAL ITCH

For symptomatic relief of anal itching, first follow the rules on page 186–87.

For anal cleansing while you are troubled with the itch, never use soap or toilet paper. Use the following instead:

Balneol (Rowell)

Directions for use are on the container.

For added relief of the itching, use either of the following every three or four hours and after each bowel movement:

Hytone Cream 0.5% (Dermik)
Vioform Cream 3% (Ciba)

For persistent, unbearable itching, see your dermatologist.

ROSACEA

Rosacea is a chronic skin disorder that is distinguished by flushing of the face, by acne-like pimples and pustules, and by small thin veins that course over the skin of the cheeks and nose.

It is typically a problem of middle-aged women after menopause, but when men blossom forth with rosacea, cosmetically disagreeable complications can arise (see below). Light complexion and blue eyes seem to predispose to rosacea.

The rash of rosacea, resembling the acne pimples of teenagers, is usually symmetrically distributed over the forehead, cheeks, nose, chin, rims of ears, and can involve the eyelids.

While the cause of rosacea is an enigma, we do know that various stimuli—hot and spicy foods, alcoholic beverages, coffee, increased environmental temperature, and even emotional tension—can lead to a dilatation, a widening, of the blood vessels of the face, resulting in exaggeration of the normal flush response. This repeated flushing and blushing is followed by permanent redness. In advanced cases, unsightly pimples, pustules, and fine veins will materialize.

Rosacea is occasionally associated with gastrointestinal disturbances, and often there is a small mite (Demodex folliculorum) that thrives and multiplies in the oil glands of the skin that seems to be implicated in many of these pustular infections.

In long-standing, severe cases, a cosmetic disfigurement of the nose—rhinophyma—can develop. This condition is especially pronounced in elderly males. The nose becomes enlarged, the tissue becomes soft, and the openings of the oil glands become widened and plugged with a cheese-like material. The classic example of rhinophyma is the bulbous nose of the late W. C. Fields.

The treatment of rosacea aims at eliminating all stimuli that encourage the widening of the superficial blood vessels of the face:

- No alcoholic beverages
- No spicy foods

- No very hot foods or drinks
- No coffee
- No seafood or pork products
- No exposure to heat or cold

While most dermatologists advise against sun exposure, some of my patients seem to benefit from moderate and careful exposure to the sun.

Dermatologists treat rosacea with either tetracycline or Accutane (oral medications requiring a prescription) as well as with various types of surface remedies.

If left untreated, rosacea may gradually increase in severity and can last for years.

TREATING ROSACEA

For mild cases of rosacea, wash with the following soap:

Fostex Cake (Westwood)

At bedtime, apply this mild mild benzoyl peroxide preparation:

Clear by Design (SmithKline)

For excessive dryness that may develop, apply the following in a thin layer whenever necessary:

Hytone Cream 0.5% (Dermik)

SPORTS-RELATED SKIN DISORDERS
[Skin Problems for Athletes]

All of us Americans seem to have at least one favorite sports activity—jogging, cycling, tennis, swimming, skiing, backpacking, mountain climbing—you name it. With so many active people, it's not surprising that there are frequent injuries and illnesses related to sports.

As healthy as exercise is, certain hazards go along with it, including the increased possibility of direct injury to your skin. You also expose yourself to many contagious skin diseases in the locker room, on gym mats, and from direct contact with infected people. And, finally, from the sweating, friction and stress you may put yourself through, you create the ideal environment for new skin conditions to develop or for existing ones to get worse.

From acne to sun poisoning, from herpes to "jogger's nipples," from "turf toe" to "bikini bottom," the competitive and weekend athlete alike risk a line-up of skin problems. But you can prevent or lessen these with proper care.

Let's look at some of these sports-related skin troubles. You'll find many of these conditions described in other chapters of this book.

190

BOXING, WRESTLING AND OTHER CLOSE CONTACT SPORTS

Anytime you have close contact with another person, you expose yourself to possible bacterial and viral infections. One common hazard of close contact sports is *impetigo*, a highly contagious bacterial infection you can get from infected opponents as well as from dirty gym mats. Impetigo gets a foothold on damaged skin, a common result of the friction and scraping from wrestling and other contact sports.

Boils are bacterial infections of the hair follicle. These painful, shiny, bright-red swellings of the skin usually develop over the elbows, forearms and knees after a bruise or break in the skin. You should see a physician if you think you have boils.

Herpes simplex infections and *dimple warts* are viral infections frequently associated with contact sports. Herpes simplex infections are so common in wrestlers that they're sometimes called "herpes gladiatorum." The highly contagious dimple warts (molluscum contagiosum) also plague wrestlers, spreading easily in the warm, moist areas caused by heavy sweat.

And, if infections aren't enough, close contact sports also increase the risk of *scabies*, a very contagious and terribly itchy infestation. Scabies mites can live on dirty gym mats and on the bodies of your opponents.

Finally, close contact sports encourage a variety of other attacks on your skin including *cuts, bruises, lacerations, abrasions* and *mat burns.*

FOOTBALL, BASEBALL, HOCKEY AND OTHER TEAM SPORTS

Some team sports create special problems because of the combination of rough activity and tight-fitting and bulky padding and uniforms.

"Acne mechanica," an infection of hair follicles where the concentration of oil glands is high, results from the rubbing, pressure, heat and sweating caused by bulky sports equipment, football helmets, catcher's masks, and heavy protective padding. Also by performing bench presses.

Boils are another common problem of team players because of frequent skin injuries and the warm, moist conditions these infections love to grow in.

Turf toe and *turf burns* are unique skin problems caused by playing on artificial turf. Turf toe appears as red, swollen and painful big toes that result from playing alternately on natural and artificial surfaces. Turf burns are abrasions that scrape off part of the skin, usually over the elbows, forearms and knees.

SWIMMING AND OTHER WATER SPORTS

Long distance swimmers often suffer from a bacterial infection called *swimmer's ear*. Exposure to water for a long time dissolves the normal oils in the ear canals, softening and weakening the tissues. Unfriendly bacteria can multiply and cause itching, swelling, pain, tenderness and a yellowish discharge from the ear. *Dimple warts* are also a common problem in swimmers.

Bikini bottom is a mild infection of the skin that results from wearing a wet bathing suit. This annoying infection frequently shows up when the sweat pores become clogged, trapping the bacteria that usually live on the skin in friendly and harmless numbers. Unable to escape, the trapped germs begin to proliferate, spread and cause trouble.

Blonds who swim a lot in pools may find that their hair has turned green! This startling color change is due to copper additives used in swimming pools. Peroxide bleaching solutions will return the hair to its normal color.

RUNNING AND JOGGING

A common problem for runners and joggers are *plantar warts*, warts on the soles of the feet. The warm, moist condition of running shoes encourages the growth of the virus that causes these warts. *Corns* are another problem of joggers. These are often caused by improperly fitting shoes, especially those that are too narrow.

Jogger's toe, also known as *tennis toe*, is another complaint of joggers, runners, tennis players and mountain climbers. Appearing as a bruise beneath the toenails, usually on the big toes, this harmless discoloration is caused by ill-fitting shoes and sudden stops which force the toes into the front of the shoe, bending the nails and breaking the blood vessels. Soft, comfortable shoes with plenty of room and trimming the toenail straight across, can prevent this problem of "short stops."

Jogger's nipples is an uncomfortable problem that can affect both sexes. It's an injury caused by friction in women who run without wearing bras and in men who jog in cotton T-shirts. The nipples become sore and red and may even bleed. To prevent this annoying condition, coat your nipples with Vaseline and wear a bra or shirt with a smooth, hard finish, such as those made of silk or semi-synthetic fabrics.

GYMNASTICS, AEROBICS AND DANCING

Gymnasts, dancers and others who do heavy stretching activity commonly develop *stretch marks*. These are thin scars that show up when the skin is distended or stretched over a long period of time. They are *not* a sign of disease.

Gymnasts may also suffer from *warts* on their palms and fingers. This common viral infection can spread from contact with gym mats, parallel bars and other gymnastics equipment.

OUTDOOR SPORTS

Direct exposure to the sun or rays reflected off snow, sand and water can create skin problems for both summer and winter athletes. *Sunburn* and *sun-poisoning* are common in baseball and tennis players, golfers, mountain climbers, swimmers and skiers. For skiers and mountain climbers, it's important to remember that the effects of ultraviolet light are stronger at higher altitudes. Taking medications, such as antibiotics or tranquilizers, may increase your risk of sunburn or sun-poisoning. To prevent sun-related skin problems year round, always apply protective sunscreens before you go out in the sun.

Warm weather athletes are often pestered by *insect bites and stings*. Make sure to pack a good, protective insect repellent in your sports bag—and use it!

Winter sports carry the added risk of *frostbite* from exposure to extreme cold. Wearing several layers of thin clothing, rather than one or two heavier layers, can help prevent frostbite. Also, because natural skin oil offers some protection to the skin, wait to shave and wash your face *after* you've come in from cold weather.

Skiers frequently suffer from *dry, chapped skin* caused by winter's low temperatures and low relative humidity.

GENERAL SPORTS ACTIVITIES

Heavy sweating, heat and tight-fitting clothing go along with many sports activities and play a part in softening and weakening the upper layers of the skin that normally protect us against the invasion and spread of harmful microorganisms—bacteria, viruses, fungi, and the scabies mite.

Athlete's foot is the infection most clearly associated with sports. Caused by a fungus, this mildly contagious disorder spreads where there is heavy sweating and poor foot hygiene. It's a frequent visitor in locker rooms, shower stalls and other warm, moist surroundings where bare feet tread.

Jock itch is a common infection of the groin caused by a fungus or yeast. Like athlete's foot, it's related to sweating and warm, moist environments.

Allergic rashes are troublesome to all types of athletes and can be caused by many natural or manufactured products: plants (poison ivy), clothing (shoes, gloves), and sports equipment (leather grips of racquets and golf clubs, basketballs, bar bells, wet suits and rubber diving masks, Fiberglas in hockey sticks, gym mats, adhesive tape, etc.). Sweating always makes these allergic rashes worse.

Heat, perspiration, friction, sun exposure and the emotional stress of competitive sports can cause or aggravate many skin problems. *Acne*, for example, is worsened by the pressure and friction of the face masks, helmets and the bulky padding of football uniforms. *Eczema* flares up with heat, perspiration and emotional stress. *Hives* can be provoked by heavy exercise, quick changes in body temperature, and stress.

In addition, athletic activities expose you to a whole batch of skin injuries. Wearing new or poorly-fitting shoes, and subjecting your feet to friction and pressure they're not used to, can quickly lead to *friction blisters* on your feet and toes. These can be treated by letting your feet rest, keeping them dry, wearing two pairs of socks, each of a different fabric, and using a foot powder.

Slamming your feet down can cause a pinching type of injury called *black heel*. As its name says, this condition appears as a black patch over the heel caused by small hemorrhages or bleeding in the upper layers of the skin, often causing concern that it might be a malignancy. It occurs almost exclusively in teenagers who play hard surface sports (basketball, tennis, handball and squash) and it disappears without treatment.

Callus formation, particularly on the feet, is the most common mechanical injury in athletes. Calluses, and their close cousins *corns*, are the skin's natural reaction to repeated rubbing and friction. These firm, thickened patches develop at points of pressure, especially over bony spots such as your heels. Gymnasts, oarsmen, golfers and tennis players often develop them on their hands. You can treat calluses by reducing the friction or pressure with pads, wraps or orthopedic appliances.

Ingrown toenails are often found on the big toes of many

athletes and result from poorly-fitting or tight shoes and poor hygiene.

Even though athletes can always expect injuries, including those to the skin, there's no reason to be fearful about participating in competitive or recreational sports. You can prevent trouble by practicing good hygiene (soap and water!), wearing clothing and sports equipment that fit properly, and protecting yourself from the sun, intense cold and insects. Remember that the best offense is a good defense. Protect your skin.

THE SKIN
OF YOUR FEET

When we gaze into a mirror, what usually gets most of our attention? I'll tell you. Our face, our eyes, our hair, and often our figure. We almost never look down at those faraway appendages that are called feet. Because, like Alice in Wonderland, who grew taller and taller while eating her cake, we say to our feet: "I'm too far away to trouble myself about you; and you must manage the best way you can." So most of us never give our feet a second thought—unless they itch, burn, or hurt.

Our foot is actually an intricate structure designed for strength and flexibility. Each foot contains 28 bones, 107 ligaments, 33 joints, and 20 muscles. With each step, an entire network of muscles, bones, and tissues, from toe to calf, goes to work to get our body moving. And moving it does: the average person will walk about 120,000 miles in his or her lifetime—more than four times the circumference of the earth.

Our feet suffer harsher treatment than any other portion of our anatomy: they bear the weight of our body, they pound the pavement, and they spend most of our waking hours stuffed into dark, tight shoes. And although they take decades of punishing service, our feet serve us admirably. They propel us through life, providing balance, support, and motion.

Encasing this highly capable, sensitive marvel of design is the skin of the foot. Different from the skin on any other part of the body, the sole of the foot is fifteen times thicker than the skin of the face and three times thicker than the skin of the palm.

While we trap our feet all day in shoes that don't permit them to "breathe," the 250,000 sweat glands continue to pour out about a half pint of perspiration every day. Inside a pair of shoes, feet swelter in a tropical environment with 80-degree heat and 80 percent humidity, making an ideal breeding ground for microorganisms: bacteria, viruses, and fungi. (The toewebs possess 1,000 times the number of bacteria that can be found on other portions of the skin.)

As we get older, our feet begin to lose their natural resilience; heel pain is common because the fat padding of the sole begins to wear thin; and the skin of the feet becomes thinner and loses some of its elasticity. Proper foot care for the elderly is essential. Healthy feet allow older people the opportunity to remain physically active and independent.

BASIC FOOT CARE FOR COMFORT AND BEAUTY

A beautiful foot, and there are beautiful feet, is one that feels supple, exhibits soft heels, has smooth toenails, has no odor, and displays no corns or calluses.

Here is how to make the skin of our feet look and feel great:

- Use good daily hygiene. That means washing your feet daily using an antibacterial soap.
- Always dry your feet and toewebs thoroughly.
- Use a medicated foot powder.
- Wear cotton socks, if possible.
- Wear shoes that fit.
- Soak feet for twenty to thirty minutes at the end of the day in warm water using special bath crystals.
- After drying, massage your feet with a foot cream.
- Trim toenails straight across to prevent ingrown nails.
- Treat your feet to an occasional pedicure.

SKIN CONDITIONS
OF THE FEET

DRY SKIN
    Even though feet perspire and lose about half a pint of fluid
each day, the moisture released from the sweat glands can evaporate quickly. Environmental factors, such as low relative humidity
and extremes of heat and cold, can dry out the skin, as can frequent
bathing with harsh soaps. When moisture is lost, the outer,
protective layer of the skin loses its flexibility and becomes dry and
brittle. About seven out of ten adult women complain of rough, dry
skin on their feet and legs, a phenomenon that is more common in
the wintertime.
    To prevent dry skin of the feet, pamper them regularly. After a
long day, soak your feet in warm water for about 30 minutes to
soothe and re-moisturize them. Adding bath crystals made especially for the feet will help soften not only the upper layers of the
skin but any corns and calluses you may have.
    After soaking, pat your feet dry with a soft towel and remove
any dry, flaky residue with a pumice stone or callus file. Then
gently massage a moisturizing cream that is specifically designed
to penetrate the thick skin of the sole and that will enhance the
skin's ability to absorb moisture.

CRACKED HEELS
    More than 18 million adults—and one in every seven women—
suffer from cracked, painful heels. This is a result of excessively dry
skin, the heels being especially susceptible to cracking because
there are continually subjected to friction and pressure.
    To relieve painful cracked heels, soak your feet for thirty
minutes in a moisturizing bath as described above, pat dry, and
then apply a soothing, emollient foot cream, such as Cracked Heel
Relief Cream, that will soften the heels, allay the pain and help
prevent infection.

ATHLETE'S FOOT
    Athlete's foot is discussed on page 171.

WARTS
    Warts are discussed on page 46.

CORNS AND CALLUSES

Corns and calluses are common foot problems. Characterized by layers of compacted dead skin cells, these protective mechanisms of the skin develop as a result of abnormal and prolonged friction and pressure between the shoe—often a tight or ill-fitting one—and the skin.

CORNS

Beginning as red, irritated skin over an underlying bony prominence, these painful and unsightly, cone-shaped areas of thickened skin are among the most common ailments to which the human foot is subject. Pressure of these hard, conical masses on sensitive nerve endings causes the pain and tenderness.

Depending upon where the corn is located, it is either hard or soft. In general, corns on the top of the toes are hard; those between the toes are soft.

Hard corns are indicative of concentrated pressure over the toes and sole of the foot, the result of deformity or dysfunction of the foot or toes. The hard, central core of these corns is often embedded in surrounding callus.

Soft corns form between the toes, almost exclusively in the fourth webspace (the last toeweb), as a result of pressure of the joint of one toe pressing against the other. The characteristic softness of these growths is due to the retention of moisture, mainly sweat which, as a result of the close proximity of the toes, is unable to evaporate.

TREATING CORNS

The first step in eliminating hard corns is to remove the cause of rubbing and friction. Wear properly fitting shoes or stretch the toe of the shoe. For immediate relief, cut off that portion of the shoe at the point where the pressure is greatest.

At the first sign of redness, use moleskin to provide protection for the affected areas. Soak feet in a foot bath with special foot bath crystals, use a corn file to remove the rough, dry skin and apply corn remover pads to ease the painful pressure.

To treat, and prevent, soft corns, keep the toewebs separated with lamb's wool at all times, and dust on a foot powder. By reducing the pressure that was responsible for the corn in the first place, these growths usually disappear by themselves.

CALLUSES

A callus is a thickened mass of skin that can form on any portion of the body. Like corns, calluses develop to protect sensitive skin from continued friction and pressure.

Calluses on the hands are very common and often indicate the type of work one does. Calluses on the bottom and sides of the feet arise where weight-bearing pressures of the body are concentrated. These calluses are hard, dry, horny-like masses of yellowish skin. Unlike corns, they do not have a central core. As the calloused skin thickens and hardens, it begins to press on sensitive nerve endings, causing pain and discomfort.

TREATING CALLUSES

The solution to the treatment and prevention of calluses of the feet is simple. Wear shoes that fit properly. Shoes should be wide enough so that the foot can expand to its full width.

Redistributing the weight evenly over the entire ball of the foot using cushioned pads made of felt or foam rubber is a popular method used in relieving and preventing callus formation.

For the long-standing calluses, there are special foot bath soaks, callus files, callus cushions and removers, and other products especially designed for these thickened and oftentimes painful masses.

All the products I mentioned in this chapter are available in the footcare sections of many drugstores and mass-merchandising outlets.

TUMORS
OF THE SKIN

A tumor is a swelling or new growth.

Tumors, which are mistakenly thought to be only malignant, include a wide variety of growths, both benign (friendly) and malignant (unfriendly), that can affect any organ of the body.

Benign tumors of the skin include warts, moles, skin tags, seborrheic keratoses, and molluscum growths. Common malignant skin tumors include the epitheliomas (carcinomas) and the malignant melanoma.

Almost everyone will develop a skin tumor in his or her lifetime, but since the great majority of skin tumors are benign and are of little consequence, people rarely bring these to the attention of the physician.

MOLES

A mole, or "nevus," is a benign (friendly) tumor of the skin. Almost everybody has at least one mole. In fact, the average number of moles on the adult human body is about forty.

Moles are usually brown or brownish-black, but they may be

skin-colored or pink or tan or even blue-black. They may be flat or raised, round or oval, single or in groups, smooth or warty, hairless or hairy. They can vary in size and shape from a fraction of an inch in diameter to huge, irregular areas covering half the body.

We don't know what causes these tumors, but we do know that they run in families and that their presence is determined even before you are born. In other words, if your parents have (or had) moles, chances are that you will, too. What these moles will look like and where they'll occur, however, seems to be a quirk of fate.

Moles that appear at birth often are called, quite appropriately, "birthmarks." The so-called strawberry mark (known medically as a hemangioma) is one of the most common. It manifests itself as a blood blister of varying size and may appear almost anywhere on the body. Another common type of birthmark is the port-wine stain (nevus flammeus), a flat, reddish-purple mark which appears most often on the back of the neck and on the face. Some birthmarks fade after three or four years. Others last a lifetime.

Most moles develop about the time of puberty or adolescence. They grow rapidly over a period of years and then slowly disappear, as if fading into the skin, in old age. Surprisingly, people in their seventies and eighties have very few moles.

The fashionable mole of a bygone era was a fortuitous happenstance. Strategically located on a woman's cheek, people considered it a sign of beauty, and the name "beauty mark" still is heard today. Jean Harlow and Marilyn Monroe had moles. Elizabeth Taylor, Telly Savalas, and Madonna have moles.

Other people, however, don't share this admiration for their own moles and seek to have them removed. The usual method for removing small moles is cutting them out under local anesthesia, a relatively simple and quick office procedure.

Although moles are harmless, they may change and become darker, causing concern. This can be due to exposure to the sun and to certain types of medications, such as cortisone. Hormone changes during puberty and pregnancy also may cause moles to become larger and darker and may even cause new ones to appear. More often than not, these changes are no cause for alarm. On rare occasions, however, changes in a mole can indicate a melanoma, the dreaded "black cancer." Although the most dangerous and fatal of all skin cancers, melanomas have an excellent cure rate if recognized early and followed by complete and wide excision.

So, if your mole suddenly becomes larger, changes in color or in texture, bleeds or crusts, or becomes itchy or painful, consult your dermatologist at once. Your doctor may recommend that the tumor be excised completely, or he or she may opt to surgically remove a small piece of tissue (known as a biopsy) and have it examined microscopically to determine the nature and extent of the apparent change. Most likely, your lesion will prove to be benign, but only a doctor can give you this reassurance.

KERATOSES

Keratoses are tumors of the skin that occur in most people in the latter decades of life.

There are two kinds of keratoses, the most common being the harmless seborrheic keratoses. These are light-brown, greasy, slightly-raised growths that chiefly involve the face, chest, and back. They are slow-growing, loosely attached to the skin, and are usually covered by a waxy-looking crust. They may be single or multiple and are usually round or oval, although they may appear in any shape. They vary in size from a fraction of an inch in diameter to up to half-dollar size or larger.

Some dermatologists call these "delayed birthmarks." Others are not so kind and refer to them as the "barnacles of old age."

Seborrheic keratoses appear to run in families. Unlike moles, they become more numerous with advancing age. They are not infectious or contagious, and they never become malignant. Many people are fond of scraping these warty growths off with their fingernails—a habit that I do not recommend. They may become infected, and they invariably grow back if not completely destroyed.

There are no internal remedies, either curative or preventive, and no salves or ointments that will rid a person of these warty growths. For cosmetic reasons, some people choose to have them removed.

Actinic keratoses, on the other hand, are very early skin cancers. And the offender in all cases are the harmful rays of the sun. Also called solar or senile keratoses, these tumors usually arise over the sun-exposed portions of the body—face, ears, forearms, neck, bald scalp, and backs of hands. They are commonly found in fair-haired, blue-eyed, fair-skinned people habitually exposed to the sun: the farmer, the sailor, the fisherman, the cattleman, the lifeguard. Black people rarely develop actinic keratoses.

These tumors are rough, dry, reddish-brown, dirty-looking growths that are firmly planted in the skin surface. If not treated, some of these may, after many years, undergo serious malignant degeneration—in other words, become cancerous. When this happens, there is the danger of the disorder spreading to lymph glands and internal organs. Therefore, it is advisable to have these tumors removed before they degenerate into malignant lesions.

Your physician can remove keratoses by any of the following methods:

- *Electrosurgery.* After the lesion has been anesthetized, the physician burns it with an electric current and then scrapes it off with a round knife (dermal curette). Bleeding is minimal, and the entire procedure takes but a few minutes.
- *Curettage.* Following a local anesthetic, the lesion is scraped off in the same manner as described above, except there is no burning. Very small lesions may be destroyed by this method even without anesthesia, but this procedure is usually reserved for stoics.
- *Liquid nitrogen cryotherapy.* This extremely cold substance (minus 320° F) is applied to the keratoses for a few seconds with a cotton applicator or a spray-type device. Over the next few days, the areas blister and the lesions are lifted up and pushed out. There is only minimal discomfort, and the cosmetic results are excellent.

A physician can treat a dozen or more of these tumors by any of these methods (depending upon the size and location) without great inconvenience to the patient.

In addition, there is a chemical substance—5-fluorouracil [5FU]—which, when locally applied for a period of a month, selectively picks out the "disagreeable" cells of the more sinister actinic keratoses. This 5FU produces a moderately severe reaction in the skin for a few weeks. Then, after the process has reached its peak, the areas slowly heal, leaving the skin smooth and soft, with no scarring. Dermatologists often recommend this procedure for multiple actinic keratoses, particularly about the face and scalp. (5FU has no effect on seborrheic keratoses.)

For those with a tendency to develop actinic keratoses—the fair-haired, blue-eyed, fair-skinned individuals—it is extremely important to avoid the sun. If your occupation or hobby requires sun exposure, always use a sunscreen such as PreSun 39.

SKIN CANCER

Malignant tumors of the skin are the most common cancers of the human body. They are also the easiest form of malignancy to treat. Almost one hundred percent of all skin cancers—there are more than 500,000 new cases diagnosed each year—are completely curable.

Since the skin is the largest and most exposed organ of the body, it is vulnerable to more environmental attacks from injury, weather, and sunlight than other organs. This, coupled with exposure of the skin to various chemicals and industrial compounds, such as tar and arsenic, predispose our large "envelope" to malignant growths.

And because these tumors are directly visible and easily accessible, they offer a unique opportunity for early diagnosis, treatment, and cure.

While the cause of skin cancer, like all cancers, remains a mystery, we do know a fair amount concerning the nature of the disease. Cancer of the skin occurs most frequently in fair-haired and fair-skinned people—those who lack adequate quantities of melanin, a pigment substance that filters out the deleterious rays of the sun. Most skin cancers develop on surfaces exposed to the sun. It is a common disease of farmers, sailors, fishermen, and athletes who often spend a lifetime outdoors.

There are two common types of skin malignancies: the basal cell carcinoma and the squamous cell carcinoma.

The basal cell carcinoma (also called basal cell epithelioma), the least aggressive of all cancers of the skin, grows very slowly and almost never spreads (metastasizes) to distant areas of the body. In its most common form it is characterized by a pearly, waxy-looking nodule which may ulcerate after a period of time. It is what I call a "friendly" malignancy and is completely curable if destroyed before extensive growth has materialized. When left untreated, these slow-growing tumors invade and destroy the adjacent and deeper tissues.

The squamous cell carcinoma (also called squamous cell epithelioma), on the other hand, is a relatively dangerous tumor, which, if allowed to grow, can spread to involve the nearby lymph glands and internal organs. Fortunately, these cancers, which occur primarily on the sun-exposed areas of the face, ears, neck, and hands, are much rarer than the basal cell type.

Early recognition and prompt, adequate treatment for all malignancies of the skin are essential. Early signs include any new growth that does not heal or any *change* in an existing growth. If you have either of these signs, see your physician at once.

If your dermatologist suspects "unfriendly" cells, he or she will surgically remove—under local anesthesia—a small piece of diseased tissue and have it examined microscopically for any possibility of malignancy. This procedure is known as a biopsy.

If the tumor is malignant, treatment will depend upon the location and size of the growth, the nature of the cancerous cells, and whether any spread is apparent. For the small, simple, "friendly" basal cell cancers, cauterization with an electric needle or surgical excision are simple, quick, and safe procedures that can be performed in the doctor's office. Other methods include freezing techniques, locally applied chemicals which selectively eradicate the malignant cells, X-ray therapy, and the new laser treatments. Regardless of the type of therapy, healing is a slow process and scarring is an inevitable consequence.

In all cases and by whatever means, the physician must completely destroy or remove the entire tumor. Periodic follow-up by your physician is necessary to insure against any recurrence of the lesion.

To prevent skin cancers, fair-skinned and sun-sensitive people should avoid unnecessary and excessive sun exposure. At the same time, *everyone* should use commercial sunscreens, with a sun-protection factor (SPF) of at least 15, to filter out the harmful and cancer-producing rays of the sun.

It's never too early, or too late, to stop this "quiet epidemic of the 20th century."

MELANOMA

Evidence from many sources suggests a steadily rising incidence of malignant melanoma in the past few decades accompanied by a rising death rate. The mortality rate in the United States from this lethal tumor is now over 6,000 a year, accounting for most of the deaths from skin cancer.

What is this malignant growth that seems to appear suddenly

out of nowhere and quickly invades not only adjoining tissue but distant organs, spreading via the blood and lymph channels?

Malignant melanomas are usually black lesions of the skin that arise in a pre-existing, dark, hairless mole—hence the epithet "black cancer." While occurring primarily on the skin surface, melanomas, which can also be pale and nonpigmented, can appear in the eye, on mucous membranes, and elsewhere. No portion of the body and no organ is immune from this deadly tumor.

Unlike the other cancers of the skin—the basal-cell and squamous-cell carcinomas—the melanoma has a striking tendency to spread to other parts of the body. Once melanoma cells extend to vital organs, they are much more difficult to treat.

While it can develop at any age, melanoma is seen most commonly in people between forty and seventy. It will strike about 30,000 men and women in the United States this year. And the risk of melanoma is expected to increase dramatically in the future.

No one has as yet discovered a single cause for melanoma, but some of the following factors appear to play a role:

- There is a higher incidence of malignant melanoma in summer climates.
- Many dermatologists believe that excessive sun exposure at an early age, and severe blistering sunburns at any age, will predispose to malignant melanoma.
- There is a greater frequency in whites because they do not have the superior unltraviolet screening capacity provided by black skin.
- People who develop melanoma are likely to have light-colored eyes, light complexions, light hair color and seem to sunburn easily.
- Although melanomas are uncommon in blacks, they can arise on the more lightly pigmented portions of the skin: the palms, soles, the nail beds, and mucous membranes of the mouth.
- If your parents, children, or siblings have had a melanoma, you have a much greater risk of developing one.
- More melanomas develop on the legs of women than men. This phenomenon is attributed to the greater exposure to sunlight as a result of women's habit of dress.
- Women taking oral contraceptives run a far greater risk of developing these black cancers than those women who have never taken birth control pills.

- Injury may also play a role in the development of melanoma. In the barefooted African Bantu, melanoma of the
  sole is more prevalent than in those who wear shoes, and in
  Ugandans the most common site of melanoma is on the sole.

Bleak as this picture is, malignant melanoma can be cured
surgically in over fifty percent of cases. The key to success is
prompt therapy. One can never be certain, however, that a melanoma has actually been cured, particularly those tumors that have
penetrated the lower layers of the skin and subcutaneous tissue
and have spread to involve the lymph glands.

How do you know whether to worry about existing moles?
Suspect a mole if it had undergone any change in size, shape, color,
or texture. The A, B, C, D danger signs of melanoma are as follows:

A. Asymmetry. If one half of a mole is unlike the other half.
B. Border irregularity. A scalloped or poorly circumscribed
   border should alert one.
C. Color varies from one area to another. Look for shades of
   red, white, or blue. Black should make one suspicious.
D. Diameter is larger than a quarter of an inch.

Moles that itch, crust, bleed, change texture or ulcerate also
point to a possible malignant change. See your physician at once if
you notice any of these changes. He or she will more than likely
recommend surgical excision of the worrisome mole followed by
microscopic analysis of the tissue.

PROBLEMS
OF THE
AGING SKIN

"A good leg will fall, a straight back will stoop, a black
    beard will turn white, a curl'd pate will grow bald, a
    fair face will wither. . . ."

Shakespeare: Henry V, Act V, scene ii, 168

An increasing proportion of our population are living longer,
and as we mature the consequences of time being to show. The
skin, hair and nails undergo characteristic changes with advancing
age, dermatologic complaints increase steadily, and most people in
their fifties and sixties have multiple skin problems, many of
which are chronic.

The importance of appearance in older people can alter their
outlook, influence their self-perception, and affect their interper-
sonal relationships. Certain components of the normal skin aging
are operating throughout life and, as yet, we have been unable to
slow these changes. A significant degree of skin aging, however, is
the end result of cumulative damage due to sun exposure.

It has recently been shown that it might be possible to reverse
some of these degenerative processes. Experimental studies have

209

indicated that the application of topical retinoic acid—Retin-A—might result in eliminating some of the fine lines and wrinkles that have been caused by overexposure to the sun.

Dermatologists and plastic surgeons have been using injectable collagen implants—a simple, in-office procedure whereby the physician injects a modified bovine collagen into the upper layers of the dermis—to reduce these cosmetically-unacceptable facial lines. Especially amenable to this type of therapy are the wrinkles of the forehead, the folds at the sides of the nose, and the area between the eyebrows. Unfortunately, the effect of this procedure is not permanent and injections must be repeated anywhere from six months to two years later. This, nonetheless, offers a satisfactory spot treatment to specific areas of the face in those otherwise unwilling or unable to undergo more aggressive surgical procedures.

Aging skin undergoes alterations in structure and function which significantly modify its appearance, and while these problems are often medically insignificant and are not life threatening, they are of profound cosmetic concern and detract from the quality of life for many older people.

Loss of elasticity, reduction in fat and moisture, changes in the supporting bone structure and muscles, wrinkles and increased dryness of the skin, changes in coloration, loss of scalp hair and growth of facial hair, and the emergence of skin growths are but a few of the many changes that eventuate with advancing years.

STRUCTURAL CHANGES IN THE AGING SKIN

The normal, "young" epidermis—the upper layer of the skin—furnishes a hardy, flexible barrier that prevents excessive water loss and provides protection from an assortment of environmental insults.

In the aging skin, certain changes in the epidermis occur. Some of these are:

1. An overall thinning of the epidermis due to reduced hormone levels. This thinning is especially noted in the areas of sun exposure and results in the thin, shiny appearance of aged skin.
2. A dwindling of the moisture content of the skin and a reduction in the oiliness of the skin surface. This leads to dryness and roughness of the skin.

3. A reduction in the protective barrier properties of the skin resulting in easily-induced irritant reactions.

4. A decrease in the number of pigment cells in both exposed and non-exposed areas. This results in irregular, mottled pigmentation and the inability to tan as deeply or as evenly as in earlier years.

5. Changes in the function of these pigment cells in sun-exposed areas induce "age spots" and patches of brown pigmentation on the neck of older women.

6. In addition, there will be an increase of benign and malignant skin tumors: seborrheic keratoses, actinic keratoses, skin cancers, and other lesions. (I have dealt with these subjects in earlier chapters.)

The function of the dermis, the lower layer of the skin, is to provide a tough matrix to support the many structures—blood vessels, nerves, appendages—that are embedded in it. Comprised chiefly of collagen and elastic fibers, the components that give the skin its texture and suppleness, the dermis decreases in thickness and density after the age of twenty, more so in females whose dermis is thinner than that of males.

In the aging dermis, the following occurs:

1. Collagen. The total amount of this component of the dermis decreases steadily throughout adult life. In addition, the collagen becomes frayed at the edges and there is alteration and thickening of the collagen fibers. Aggravated by sun exposure, these changes result in:

   a. Skin deterioration. The skin becomes more mobile and is easily picked up and pinched into folds. This is commonly observed over the tops of the hands. The skin becomes fragile and is easily torn, and wound healing is delayed.

   b. Permanent widening and tortuosity of the superficial capillaries which are seen conspicuously over the nose and cheeks.

   c. Black-and-blue marks. Loss of collagen support to the blood vessels make them susceptible to rupture by even the slightest trauma. Large discolored areas result from minor knocks, particularly over the tops of the hands and forearms where the skin has already been damaged by sun exposure.

   2. Elastic Fibers. As the elastin network ages, the elastic fibers thicken and degenerate, resulting in:

      a. Wrinkles. The loss of elastic fibers, coupled with changes in the collagen, leads to fine wrinkles initially observed over the outer part of the eyes ("crow's feet"), forehead, and other sun-exposed areas. Additional factors that contribute to wrinkles include the person's facial expressions ("the woman who doesn't smile never gets wrinkles"), the position in which the person sleeps, and whether the individual is a smoker.

      b. Furrows develop at the site of facial expression lines. These are noted primarily over the upper lip in women and are also seen on the forehead, and the folds at the sides of the nose.

      c. Sagging and folds are commonly seen over the eyelids, neck, jaw, and arms.

      d. "Chicken neck." The skin of the sides of the neck has a ridged appearance with thickening around the openings of the hair follicles, making the skin look rippled. This phenomenon also appears over the temples and cheeks and is more common in women.

      e. "Peasant's neck." This yellowish, thick, weatherbeaten, leathery skin of the back of the neck, with deep, crisscrossing furrows, is noted in those men chronically exposed to the sun.

In addition, there is a decrease in the surface temperature of the skin. This produces skin that is pale in appearance. The small blood vessels around the appendages—sweat glands, oil glands, and hair follicles—also diminish in density resulting in decreased sweating, decreased oiliness, and thinning of the hair.

For more information on some of the procedures that are used to reduce or eradicate the signs of aging skin, consult your dermatologist.

To prevent many of the signs of aging, stay out of the sun!

ZITS

A zit is a common, colloquial expression that young people often use when referring to an acne "bump," or pimple. These acne bumps, or zits, come in many sizes, and, depending upon how large they are, can go by a variety of other names.

The common, everyday, garden-variety of zit is the one that is about the size of a pea.

A larger zit, the size of a small grape, is called a "goober." So if you have lots of zits and goobers, you usually have a face full of acne: a "pizza face."

When the goober become very large, say, the size of a large cherry, I call it a "zinger."

And then there's the "honker." This is the third eye you wake up with the morning of the prom.

Finally, we have the "screamer." This is when your mother sees you first thing in the morning with a monstrous, walnut-sized lump on your cheek and lets out a tremendous scream!

There are also "splashers," but I won't elaborate on these; you can probably guess what they are.

So now you have it: the zit, the goober, the zinger, the honker, and the screamer.

If you've read this book carefully, you should never be bothered by any of the above.

HOME REMEDIES

The following home remedies—products often found in your own cupboard or refrigerator—are sometimes very helpful in relieving the itching, pain, and discomfort of many skin ailments. Please be aware that not all of these work for everybody, and that if you have a disorder that is stubborn, prolonged, very itchy or painful for days or weeks, you should see your general physician or your dermatologist.

1. Yogurt—can be used for severe *itching* of the vulva due to *yeast infections* or to painful *cold sore* infections. Put two table-spoonfuls of unflavored yogurt on a handkerchief or sanitary napkin and apply it to the itchy or painful area and leave on for several hours. Re-apply as needed.

Also excellent for many cases of *rectal itch*.

Eating yogurt, 4 tablespoonfuls daily, can often prevent recurrent *canker sores*.

2. Tea Bags—excellent for *smelly and sweaty feet*. Take two tea bags and put them in a pint of boiling water for fifteen minutes. Then remove the tea bags and pour the pint of strong, hot tea in a basin filled with two quarts of cool water. Soak your feet for

twenty to thirty minutes daily for a week or ten days. No smell! No sweat! Repeat as often as needed.

Tea bags are also good for painful *canker sores* in the mouth. Immerse a tea bag in half a glass of tepid water until sopping wet. Remove the tea bag, squeeze out almost all the water, and then apply the tea bag directly to the canker sore and hold it there for a few minutes. You may be pleasantly surprised.

3. Lemons [fresh]—good for removing *freckles* and *age spots*. Often works as well as the expensive "fade creams." Cut a fresh lemon and squeeze the juice out of half in a small bowl. Using a cotton ball, wipe the affected spots with the lemon juice twice daily. Try this for six to eight weeks. Repeat as necessary.

4. Onions—also can be used for removing *freckles* and *age spots*. Slice a red onion in half and rub on the spot twice daily. Continue until the spot or spots fade.

Onions are also good to prevent *insect bites and stings*. Eat a couple of raw onions (great with hamburgers!) daily during the summer. The insects will usually avoid you!

5. Garlic—along with the onions, eating garlic will often prevent *mosquitoes* from attacking you.

6. Egg white—for those of you with facial *wrinkles* or large *pores*, the best and least expensive way of getting rid of them for about two hours (just before the party) is as follows:

About an hour before your party, wash your face thoroughly with a mild soap. Then beat up two egg whites into a meringue (until they are stiff). Apply the egg whites over your face and leave on for twenty to thirty minutes. Then rinse off with cool water (not hot, else you'll have scrambled eggs on your face!) and pat dry. Then put on your makeup. You'll be wrinkle free for about two hours. This is much less expensive than the 100-dollar an ounce anti-wrinkle creams, which also work for about two hours.

7. Meat tenderizer—excellent for *insect bites and stings*. For a mild bee or wasp sting, or for annoying mosquito and flea bites, make a paste of one-half teaspoon of unseasoned meat tenderizer with a few drops of water and apply directly to the bite or sting. You should obtain relief in a matter of minutes. For you outdoors people: always carry a bottle of the meat tenderizer with you when you plan a trip.

8. Ice cubes—an ice cube applied to a fresh *cold sore* will often abort the spread of the condition. Ice cubes are also good for *insect bites and stings*.

9. Adhesive tape—excellent for *warts* around and under fin-

gernails. Apply four layers of the tape—two longwise and two around the finger up to the first joint—to make it airtight. Leave on for a week. Remove for twelve hours and re-apply for another week. Keep doing this until the wart gets "tired" and disappears, leaving no mark or scar! (see page 48)

10. Nail polish—excellent for *chigger* bites. Apply the polish right on the bite and the chigger will suffocate and die.

HOW TO APPLY
COMPRESSES AND
WET DRESSINGS

For skin problems in localized areas (except hands and feet), this is the proper method to apply compresses or wet dressings:

Use either a folded cotton handkerchief or pieces of bed linen folded eight layers thick. Dip this into a prepared Bluboro solution [See page 167] and gently wring it out so that the cloth is sopping wet. Pat this on the affected area—on and off, on and off—remoistening the cloth when necessary. Do this for ten or fifteen minutes every hour or so until the rash has cooled down, has begun to dry up, or until the crusts have been removed. After compressing, pat the area dry, then apply the appropriate cream or lotion. (If you plan to use the same cloth for future compresses, make sure to rinse it out in plain water to avoid any chemical build-up.)

For acute, weeping and oozing rashes of the fingers and hands, the best way to soak these areas is as follows:

Purchase two or three pairs of Dermal Gloves from your drugstore. With the gloves on, place your hands in the Bluboro solution and remove them every five seconds—in and out, in and out. Do this for ten or fifteen minutes and then remove the gloves. Pat dry. (Never let the gloves dry on your hands!)

Repeat this procedure every hour or so until the oozing,

217

weeping, or crusting has begun to dry up. At bedtime, apply the recommended cream or lotion and wear the dry gloves to bed.

For weeping or oozing skin problems of the feet and toewebs, follow these steps:

1. Put on soft, white cotton socks. If your toes are affected, keep them separated with lamb's wool or one-inch squares of old but clean cotton sheets (do not use cotton balls).
2. Fill a one-gallon plastic tub or basin with the Bluboro solution (in proper proportions) and put your feet in. Count to five. Take the right foot out and rest it on a clean, large bath towel. Count to five. Put the right foot back into the basin. Count to five. Take the left foot out and rest it on the towel. Count to five. Put the left foot back into the basin. Count to five. Take the right foot out and rest it on the towel, etc.
3. Continue this treatment for twenty to thirty minutes. You can do this while watching TV, reading, or writing letters. (Don't do this while drying your hair or using anything electrical.) Try to keep the water warm by adding to the solution every so often. Do not let the socks dry on your feet!
4. After you have finished soaking, remove the socks and lamb's wool and dry your feet thoroughly. Do not leave them damp.
5. Repeat the entire procedure every three or four hours until the weeping and oozing have stopped.
6. At bedtime, apply the recommended cream and put on a clean, dry pair of white, cotton socks.
7. If your toewebs are affected, as in athlete's foot, always— 24 hours a day—keep your toes separated with lamb's wool or linen material until the condition clears up.

GLOSSARY

Acne. A common skin eruption that usually appears on the face, chest, and back. Commonly begins in adolescence when the oil glands enlarge and become inflamed. Characterized by blackheads, pimples, pustules, and occasionally cysts and scars.

Actinic. An adjective meaning relating or pertaining to rays or beams of light.

Allergy. A hypersensitivity to a chemical, food, drug, metal, sunlight, or other substance.

Alopecia. Hair loss

Alopecia Areata. Hair loss occurring in patches.

Androgen. A hormone that promotes male characteristics.

Antibiotic. A substance, such as penicillin and tetracycline, that stops the growth of certain germs.

Antihistamine. A chemical used to alleviate itching in allergic reactions.

Aphthous Stomatitis. Canker sores.

Ashy Skin. Grayish-looking skin in black people that is nothing more than dry skin. It is *not* a sign of disease.

Athlete's Foot. A superficial fungous infection of the feet. Also known as ringworm of the feet.

219

Atopic Dermatitis. See Eczema

Autoimmune Disease. A disease resulting from a disordered immune reaction in which antibodies are produced against one's own tissues. For example, lupus erythematosus.

Bacteria. Germs capable of producing disease.

Benign. Not malignant (noncancerous).

Blackhead. A black-tipped plug of dried oil that has blocked a pore of an oil gland.

Blister. A swelling of the upper layers of the skin filled with fluid.

Boil. A painful and tender swelling of the skin caused by various bacteria.

Canker Sores. Painful ulcers of the mouth or tongue. Also known as aphthous stomatitis.

Cellulite. A "normal abnormality" of almost all women characterized by the waffled-looking fat of the buttocks and upper thighs. It is a fancy name for plain fat. It is *not* a disease.

Cholasma. Patchy excess pigmentation. See Melasma.

Cold Sore. A small blister on the face or other portion of the body caused by the herpes virus. See herpes.

Collagen. The generic name for a family of proteins that are the major fibrous components of skin, tendons, ligaments, cartilage, and bone. It is what gives the skin its resilient and elastic quality.

Contact Dermatitis. An allergy or irritation on the skin resulting from exposure to certain substances (chemicals, plants, cosmetics, etc.).

Crabs. Pubic lice.

Cradle Cap. Seborrhic dermatitis in infancy.

Crust. A scab or dried secretion on the surface of the skin.

Cuticle. The skin that is attached to the base of the nails.

Cyst. A skin tumor, almost always benign, filled with fluid or solid matter.

Dandruff. Visible scaling of the scalp.

Depigmentation. Loss of color or pigment.

Depilatory. A substance that removes hair.

Dermatitis. Inflammation of the skin; an eczema.

Dermatosis Papulosa Nigra. Tiny, smooth, raised, mole-like spots that appear on the face and neck of black people that are darker than the surrounding skin. They never become malignant.

Diaper Rash. Any eruption on an infant's buttocks, genital and anal areas, lower abdomen, and upper thighs that appears during the diaper-wearing stage.

Dimple Wart. See Molluscum Contagiosum.

Eczema. Synonym for dermatitis. Used by the dermatologist, it means atopic dermatitis.

Electrolysis. Destruction of the hair root with an electric current.

Endocrine glands. Certain hormone-producing glands (thyroid, adrenal, etc.).

Epidermis. The outer layer of the skin.

Fever Blister. Synonym for cold sores or herpes.

Follicle. A tiny, sac-like structure out of which the hair grows.

Folliculitis. A hair follicle infection.

Freckles. Small spots of pigmentation over the face and shoulders in some people (often redheads) that get worse when exposed to the sun.

Frostbite. The sharp, painful sensations that result from severe cold injury.

Fungus. A microorganism (actually a miniature plant) that is responsible for various fungous infections (athlete's foot, jock itch, tinea versicolor, and others).

Genital Herpes. Cold sores of the genital region.

Herpes Simplex. Cold sores. An inflammation of the skin caused by a virus and characterized by small, itchy blisters on a red base. Also known as fever blisters.

Herpes Zoster. Shingles.

Hirsutism. Excessive growth of hair; hypertrichosis.

Hives. An allergic reaction characterized by itching and burning wheals (welts) on the skin.

Hyperpigmentation. Excessive coloration of the skin.

Hypersensitivity. The tendency to be allergic.

Hypertrichosis. Too much hair; hirsutism.

Hypopigmentation. Decreased coloration of the skin.

Ichthyosis. A dry, rough, scaly hereditary skin disorder. Also called "fishskin disease."

Impetigo. An infectious disease of the skin caused by the streptococcus or staphylococcus germs and characterized by "stuck-on," honey-colored crusts.

Integument. The skin.

Infestation. The invasion of the skin by a mite or parasite. Scabies and lice are infestations.

Itch. An irritation of the skin that causes a desire to scratch.

Jock Itch. An itching and inflammation of the groins, usually caused by a fungus. Also known as ringworm of the groin.

Keloid. An enlarged or overgrown scar.

Keratosis. A scaly, crusted, wart-like growth.

Keratosis Pilaris. A common rash over the backs of the arms and thighs that looks and feels like a cheese grater. It is a harmless condition and usually improves in the warmer weather.

LE. An abbreviation for lupus erythematosus.

Lice. Parasites that cause itching.

Lichen Planus. An itchy skin rash characterized by flat, violet-colored bumps that generally appear on the wrists, ankles, and lower back.

Lupus Erythematosus. A collagen disease that can involve any organ of the body. When it involves the skin, it appears as disc-shaped, red, scarred patches on the face and scalp. Same as LE.

Malignant. Cancerous.

Melanin. The brownish-black pigment produced in the skin.

Melanocyte. A cell that produces melanin.

Melanoma. A malignant tumor of the skin that spreads rapidly.

Melasma. A brownish, mottled pigmentation of the skin, usually seen on the face of women. Also know as chloasma.

Miliaria. Prickly heat.

Mite. A parasite of the skin. Scabies is caused by a mite.

Mole. A birthmark—or nevus; a pigmented growth on the skin, with or without hair.

Molluscum Contagiosum. See Dimple Wart.

Monilia. A yeast-like fungus responsible for many skin rashes, especially in the groins.

Nevus. A birthmark; a mole.

Nevus Flammeus. Port-wine stain.

Nit. The egg of a louse.

Oral. By mouth.

Paronychia. An inflammation of the soft tissue around the nails.

Pediculosis. Lice infestation.

Perleche. Cracks in the corners of the mouth.

Photosensitivity. An exaggerated sensitivity to light.

Pityriasis Rosea. A common skin disorder that begins with a solitary patch of redness and scaling and evolves over a period of about two weeks in a fairly generalized rash. It is not contagious.

Plantar Wart. A wart on the bottom of the foot.

Port-wine Stain. A flat, reddish-purple mark which appears most often on the face and on the back of the neck. Also called nevus flammeus.

Prickly Heat. A common disorder of the sweat apparatus that arises when the free flow of sweat to the surface of the skin is obstructed.

Pruritus. Itching.

Pseudofolliculitis Barbae. See Razor Bumps.

Psoriasis. A common chronic, inflammatory skin disease characterized by scaly patches.

Pustule. A pus-filled pimple.

Pyoderma. An impetigo-like infection of the skin accompanied by weeping, oozing, and painful crusts.

Rash. An eruption on the skin.

Razor Bumps. Ingrown hairs of the beard in black men. The technical name for this is pseudofolliculitis barbae.

Ringworm. A common term for a fungous infection of the skin. Athlete's foot is a ringworm infection.

Rosacea. A chronic skin disorder of middle-aged people, characterized by redness of the face accompanied by acne-like pimples and pustules.

Scabies. An intensely itchy, contagious skin condition caused by a mite.

Scar. A permanent mark left on the skin following a wound or surgical procedure.

Sebaceous gland. A gland of the skin that produces sebum (oil).

Seborrheic Dermatitis. An inflammation of the sebaceous glands producing yellow, greasy scales on the scalp and face.

Sebum. The oily material produced by the sebaceous glands.

Shingles. Herpes Zoster. A viral infection caused by a virus and characterized by itching, pain, and a rash on one side of the body.

Skin Tags. Small, fleshy growths that are often seen in the armpits and around the neck. They are benign tumors.

Stretch Marks. Very thin scars that commonly develop when the skin is stretched for a long period of time.

Tinea Versicolor. A "friendly" fungous infection of the skin characterized by fawn-colored, scaly patches over the chest and back.

Topical. Surface (as in topical medication as opposed to internal medication.)

Tumor. A new growth. A tumor can be benign (friendly) or malignant (unfriendly).

Ulcer. An open sore or wound.

Urticaria. Hives.

Vitiligo. A skin disorder characterized by patchy loss of pigment.

Wart. A contagious growth on the skin caused by a virus.

Wen. A smooth, round, dome-like, soft or moderately hard tumor of the scalp filled with greasy, cheese-like, odoriferous material.

Wheal. A welt or hive.

Whitehead. A small plug that blocks the skin pore; actually, a closed blackhead.

Zits. Common acne pimples.

INDEX

232